Medical Error

Marilynn M. Rosenthal
Kathleen M. Sutcliffe
Editors

THE UNIVERSITY OF
MICHIGAN FORUM
ON HEALTH POLICY

Medical Error

What Do We Know?
What Do We Do?

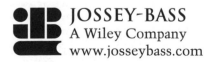

JOSSEY-BASS
A Wiley Company
www.josseybass.com

Published by

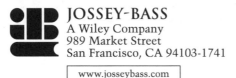

JOSSEY-BASS
A Wiley Company
989 Market Street
San Francisco, CA 94103-1741

www.josseybass.com

Jossey-Bass books and products are available through most bookstores. To contact Jossey-Bass directly, call (888) 378-2537, fax to (800) 605-2665, or visit our website at www.josseybass.com.

Substantial discounts on bulk quantities of Jossey-Bass books are available to corporations, professional associations, and other organizations. For details and discount information, contact the special sales department at Jossey-Bass.

We at Jossey-Bass strive to use the most environmentally sensitive paper stocks available to us. Our publications are printed on acid-free recycled stock whenever possible, and our paper always meets or exceeds minimum GPO and EPA requirements.

Jossey-Bass also publishes its books in a variety of electronic formats. Some content that appears in print may not be available in electronic books.

Library of Congress Cataloging-in-Publication Data

Medical error : what do we know? what do we do? / [edited by] Marilynn M. Rosenthal, Kathleen M. Sutcliffe.—1st ed.
    p. ; cm.
Includes bibliographical references and index.
  ISBN 0-7879-6395-X (alk. paper)
  1. Medical errors.
  [DNLM: 1. Medical Errors—prevention & control. 2. Malpractice. 3. Patient Satisfaction. 4. Risk Management. WB 100 M48673 2002] I. Rosenthal, Marilynn M. II. Sutcliffe, Kathleen M., 1950–
  R729.8 .M433 2002
  610—dc21

                                              2002005157

HB Printing 10 9 8 7 6 5 4 3 2   **FIRST EDITION**

Contents

Foreword

"Physician: First, do no harm" is the dictum from Hippocrates that every medical student learns and every health care professional and staff person must commit to meet.

In health care, there are many, many decisions that involve balancing benefits against risks, choices about cancer chemotherapy or x rays or exercise regimens, for example. But far too many adverse events occur in patients without benefit, due to, simply stated, mistakes. Most horrific are right-left mistakes in surgery on a limb or essential body part. Failure to protect the patient or restrain the patient, when necessary, leads to many preventable falls and subsequent injuries. Medications are a major part of the problem, due to neglect of known or knowable patient allergies, wrong drug administered, wrong dosage prescribed, or wrong dosage delivered. The Food and Drug Administration tolerates too many drugs with confusingly similar names, packaging, or labeling, leading to look-alikes and sound-alikes. Our e-mail is full of "alerts" about such medication problems (Institute for Safe Medication Practices, 2001). Medical devices may malfunction, for reasons ranging from design to application to settings to monitoring. And this list could go on.

Hospitals have long been expected to comply with extensive safety standards for their patients and their employees in order to sustain accreditation, usually by the Joint Commission on

Accreditation of Healthcare Organizations (JCAHO). Accreditation processes have become a lot stiffer in the past few years as many studies have been published showing shocking frequencies of serious errors and serious consequences. This literature was synthesized by the Institute of Medicine (IOM) Committee on Quality of Health Care in America, whose report *To Err Is Human: Building a Safer Health System* (Kohn, Corrigan, & Donaldson, 2000) generated major attention. Drawing on data from a study in Colorado and Utah and another in New York, the committee combined the percentage of patients admitted to hospitals who had an adverse event (3 to 6 percent), the proportion of those who died (7 to 14 percent), the proportion of deaths judged to have been preventable (50 percent), and the number of admissions in 1997 (34 million) to generate an estimate of 44,000 to 98,000 deaths from medical care errors in that year. That figure is greater than the number of deaths from motor vehicle injuries (43,000), breast cancer (42,000), or AIDS (16,000) in that year. And that figure does not include deaths from preventable adverse events in outpatient care, home care, or self-care.

That report and the follow-on report, *Crossing the Quality Chasm: A New Health System for the 21st Century* (Committee on Quality of Health Care in America, Institute of Medicine, 2001), led to federal action to create the Center for Patient Safety in the Agency for Healthcare Research and Quality (with a budget increase to support the center's program) and the National Quality Forum, with consumers and providers and employers as participants. Efforts to reduce error were redoubled in hospitals, health care systems, and health plans, as well as on the part of the JCAHO and the National Committee for Quality Assurance (NCQA).

The aim is to design safety into the health care system: to practice prevention. An analogy to the aviation industry is commonly drawn; in 1998, there were no deaths at all from commercial aviation in the United States (unfortunately not true in 2001). There is much to be learned about prevention from the aviation, chemical, and other industrial sectors. One important point is the need for both accountability and transparency, complex issues in a field so fearful of malpractice litigation. Quality improvement directed at the system and setting of care is gaining in emphasis, which is good. Quality assurance tied to regulatory and accreditation compliance and liability remains necessary.

At the University of Michigan Health System and at our affiliated Ann Arbor Veterans Affairs Medical Center, patient safety has had high visibility for some time. As recommended widely, and highlighted in this book, there is leadership committed to safety both for patients and for staff; an organizational culture that values, emphasizes, and publishes on the recognition of errors and the process of learning from errors; an active patient safety committee with public members; and a safety program that involves training, compliance, research studies, information system support, and root cause analysis of adverse events and near misses. Up-to-date guidance on the value of safety practices is now available (University of California at San Francisco – Stanford University Evidence-Based Practice Center, 2001).

In this book, which emerged from the conference "What Do We Know About Medical Mishaps," held at the University of Michigan Medical Center in October 1999, editors Marilynn Rosenthal and Kathleen Sutcliffe have brought together a comprehensive and constructive review of medical mishaps. Like the IOM committee, this book begins with a look at the findings of and responses to the Harvard Medical Practice Study—whose researchers generally conducted their studies outside their own institution and their own state! The contributors to this book also give major attention to behavioral and consumer-patient views. Efforts by individuals and by institutions and systems to improve the overall quality of care, measured as outcomes of all kinds, can and should begin with safety, per the Hippocratic dictum. In Crossing the Quality Chasm, the IOM describes quality health care for the patient in six dimensions: safe, effective, patient-centered, timely, efficient, and equitable. Care must also be cost effective, so safety and quality programs that control or reduce costs are especially valuable.

A forthcoming IOM committee report will carry this message forward with emphasis on the patient, beginning with the patient-centered dimension of the *Chasm* report and expanding to examine quality improvement, quality oversight, and quality research over the life span of the patient, across multiple settings and payers, and with multiple quality and safety regimens.

The two IOM reports have been invaluable in focusing national attention on issues of patient safety. However, several challenges have been raised since the reports were published. Are the data accurate? How can reliable data be collected? Are systems models from industry appropriate for clinical medicine? What is the interplay between individual and systems factors in medical adverse events and mistakes? Has there been sufficient evaluation of the various efforts, programs, and enterprises now in place to improve patient safety?

As the editors of this book conclude, the "struggle" to markedly improve care for patients is necessary, worthy, and feasible. Nothing less than our best will be credible.

Gilbert S. Omenn, M.D., Ph.D.
Executive Vice President for Medical Affairs
University of Michigan

References

Committee on Quality of Health Care in America, Institute of Medicine. (2001). *Crossing the quality chasm: A new health system for the 21st century.* Washington, DC: National Academy Press.

Institute for Safe Medication Practices. (2001). It's time for a new model of accountability. *ISMP Medication Safety Alert 2001*, 6(16), 1–2.

Kohn, L. T., Corrigan, J. M., & Donaldson, M. S. (Eds.); Committee on Quality of Health Care in America, Institute of Medicine. (2000). *To err is human: Building a safer health system.* Washington, DC: National Academy Press.

University of California at San Francisco–Stanford University Evidence-Based Practice Center. (2001). *Making health care safer: A critical analysis of patient safety practices* (Evidence Report/Technology Assessment No. 43, AHRQ Publication No. 01-E058). Rockville, MD: Agency for Healthcare Research and Quality.

Preface

This book and the multimedia health policy series of which it is a part are predicated on this central belief: challenging social problems and social policy are best understood through the juxtaposition of objective data, positions, perspectives, ideas, and ideologies. These may come from the political, organizational, institutional, social science, or historical arenas. This naturally produces a clash of perspectives: between the social scientist, the bureaucrat, the policymaker, the politician, the practitioner, and the consumer.

Our central purpose is to lay out these different views on the subject of medical error, articulated by the best people we can find. Of course editors have their own biases and preferences. We have, however, tried to put ours aside and help our audience clarify and understand varying viewpoints. We are dedicated to raising standards for information and for judging "facts," sometimes pointing out how difficult it is to establish the facts. Positions and ideologies are often based on assumptions. But often issues are so complex that assumptions are all any of us have, particularly when a set of problems demands immediate action.

Many of the papers included in this volume were presented first in a symposium at the University of Michigan, and this book reflects the symposium's commitment to juxtaposition. How else can we all understand the dynamic and confounding context within which we discuss a problem as important and complex as medical mishaps?

Of course health care organizations need to move quickly to reduce and prevent medical mishaps. They need to provide tools to health and medical practitioners. The pressures to jump at any tools are great. We believe this book will provide an informed and sensitive context within which to choose those tools with a fighting chance for success.

Medical Error: What Do We Know? What Do We Do? has five parts. Part One sets the stage with a discussion of the Harvard Medical Practice Study of 1990, which initiated the present focus on seeking ways to understand and reduce medical error, and related studies. The chapters in Part Two present both patients' and health care providers' experience of medical error and the directions in which that experience is taking us. Part Three looks at managing error from the points of view of managed care, of formal risk management, and of evidence-based medicine and outcomes research. Part Four examines systems models for reducing error that are attracting much attention. And in Part Five, we sum up the objective data, positions, perspectives, ideas, and ideologies of the contributors to this volume and, on that foundation, offer an agenda for action, research, and education.

Join us in exploring the complexities of formulating, legislating, implementing, and evaluating health policy and programs across a variety of current and pressing national concerns among which medical mishaps constitute a most pressing concern.

Our ideas have been shaped by a host of valued colleagues whose work we admire: people such as Troy Brennan, John Carroll, Liam Donaldson, Amy Edmondson, Maggie Lampert, Synneve Oregard, Jim Reason, Steve Shortell, Michal Tamuz, Charles Vincent, Merrlyn Walton, Robert Wears, Karl Weick, and Ross M. Wilson. Shelly Whitmer gave us invaluable help in formatting and organizing the materials. We also thank all the contributors for the efforts they made and for their patience with the editing process.

University of Michigan FORUMS appear in books, articles, Web sites, and journal supplements. Watch www.med.umich.edu/forum for details.

March 2002   Marilynn M. Rosenthal
                                                  Ann Arbor, Michigan

                                                  Kathleen M. Sutcliffe
                                                  Ann Arbor, Michigan

About the University of Michigan FORUM

This book is part of a multimedia health policy series called The University of Michigan FORUM. This series is predicated on the belief that social policy is best understood through the juxtaposition of positions, perspectives, ideas, and ideologies. Our central purpose is to lay out those different views, articulated by the best people we can find, and to try to help our audience and readers clarify and understand varying viewpoints. Often, positions and ideologies are based on assumptions, and sometimes issues are so complex that that is the best we can do.

Additional publications by University of Michigan FORUM will appear in book, article, website, and journal supplement forms. Visit www.med.umich.edu/psm/FORUM.html for details.

Marilynn M. Rosenthal
Professor and Director
University of Michigan FORUM on Health Policy
Ann Arbor, Michigan

The Editors

Marilynn M. Rosenthal is a professor and medical sociologist. She is associate director of the University of Michigan medical school's Program in Society and Medicine, and coordinates the University of Michigan Health Policy Forum. She is the director of the Program in Health Policy Studies at the University of Michigan in Dearborn.

Rosenthal's primary research interests involve physician self-regulation. Her grants and honors include the Danforth Fellowship for Women, University of Michigan Hopwood writing award, Swedish Visiting Scholar award, British Kings Fund Grants, Fulbright Research Award, and University of Michigan Faculty Recognition Award and Distinguished Faculty Research Award.

Her publications include nine books and over forty articles. Among the books are *Dealing with Medical Malpractice* (1988), *The Incompetent Doctor* (1997), and *Medical Mishaps: Pieces of the Puzzle* (1999). In the last year, her work related to patient safety has been quoted in a number of national magazines and articles. She has been a visiting scholar at Wolfson College, University of Oxford, and visiting lecturer at Harvard School of Public Health. She holds a Ph.D. degree from the University of Michigan.

Kathleen M. Sutcliffe is associate professor of organizational behavior and human resource management at the University of Michigan Business School. She received a B.A. degree from the University of Michigan, a B.S. degree from the University of Alaska, an M.N. degree in community health from the University of Washington, and a Ph.D. degree in management from the University of Texas at Austin. Before studying for her doctoral degree she worked as a community health nurse practitioner in a rural Alaskan community, as a health care program consultant for the State of Alaska, and as a senior manager for an Alaska Native Health Corporation, headquartered in Anchorage. Her research program has been devoted to investigating how organizations and their members cope with uncertainty and how organizations can be designed to be more reliable. Her research has appeared in numerous scholarly journals, and her co-authored book, *Managing the Unexpected: Assuring High Performance in an Age of Complexity* (with Karl E. Weick, 2001), describes how organizations achieve reliability.

The Contributors

Susan Anderson received her B.S.N. and M.S.N. degrees from Wayne State University and her M.B.A. degree from California State University. A registered nurse with experience in many areas of clinical practice, most recently in neonatal nursing, she began working in the field of risk management in 1991 and has had the honor of serving the Michigan Society of Healthcare Risk Management as director in 1998–99 and as secretary in 2000–01. She is a member of the American Society for Healthcare Risk Management and has obtained certification through the American Hospital Association in risk management. She is presently a risk management consultant for health care at the University of Michigan.

Kenneth J. Appleby received his B.A. degree in education from the University of Michigan-Dearborn. He has been actively involved in the field of health care risk management for over twenty years. He is an associate in risk management (ARM) and a certified professional in healthcare risk management (CPHRM). Currently he is director of risk management at the University of Michigan Hospitals and Health Centers.

Troyen A. Brennan is professor of medicine at Harvard Medical School and president of the Brigham and Women's Physicians Organization. He is also professor of law and public health at the

Harvard School of Public Health. Brennan received his M.D., J.D., and M.P.H. degrees from Yale University and trained in internal medicine at the Massachusetts General Hospital in Boston. His research interests are the legal and ethical issues in medicine and public health, and he is the author of over two hundred peer-reviewed articles and four books. Elected to the American Board of Internal Medicine board of directors in 1999, he serves on the Committee on Recertification and the Committee on General Internal Medicine and chairs the ABIM Foundation/ACP-ASIM Foundation/ European Society for Internal Medicine Medical Professionalism Project 2000.

Darrell A. Campbell Jr. is chief of clinical affairs at the University of Michigan Health System. He is responsible for the overall quality of care delivered in this organization and has a special interest in patient safety. He is also professor of surgery in the Department of Surgery and has for many years specialized in solid organ transplantation, particularly kidney, liver, and pancreas. He received a B.S. degree in zoology from Michigan State University and an M.D. degree from George Washington University, graduating with distinction. From 1972 through 1979, he undertook general surgery training at the University of Michigan Medical School and also spent two years as an investigator in the National Cancer Institute in the area of immunodiagnostics. Following his training, he began his special interest in transplantation. In recent years, he has also focused on the related subjects of physician wellness and patient safety, lecturing nationally on the subject of physician burnout, particularly among surgeons. Currently serving as coinvestigator on two NIH-funded grants ("Patient Safety in Surgery" and "The Effect of Health Care Working Conditions on Quality of Care"), Campbell also sits on the Executive Committee of the National Surgical Quality Improvement Program.

Theresa L. Carroll earned a B.S.N. degree from Mt. Mercy (now Carlow) College and M.S.N. and Ph.D. degrees, the latter in higher education, from the University of Pittsburgh. A registered nurse, she has held academic and administrative positions at the University of Pittsburgh and Duquesne University and is currently professor and associate dean for academic affairs at the University of Texas Health Science Center Houston School of Nursing and professor of management and policy science at the University of Texas Health Science Center Houston School of Public Health. Carroll has published extensively in the area of nursing administration and is on the editorial board of the *Nursing Administration Quarterly*. She has been awarded extramural funding to support her research on the leadership skills and attributes that women will need to succeed in the twenty-first century, nurse executive job loss, and the characteristics of nurse managers, and to develop, implement, and evaluate three nurse-managed wellness centers in two states.

Patricia L. Cornett is the founder and director of MedWrite Associates, a medical writing, editing, and publications firm begun in 1985. Before that, she was scientific publications editor at Henry Ford Hospital (Detroit) and managing editor of the *Henry Ford Hospital Medical Journal*. For nine years, she was assistant professor of technical communication at Lawrence Technological University, Southfield, Michigan, where she established a technical communication program and served as its director for three years. In her capacity as a medical writer, Cornett has edited and authored many professional publications on a wide range of health care topics, most recently the chapter "Writing Abstracts" in *Essays for Biomedical Communicators* (2001). A member of the American Medical Writers Association (AMWA) since 1978, Cornett was AMWA national president in 1988–89. She is also an experienced workshop leader, panelist, and panel moderator. She holds a Ph.D. degree in English from the University of Michigan, where her field of concentration was Shakespeare and Renaissance drama.

Margaret Copp Dawson received a B.A. degree in cultural anthropology from the University of Michigan and a B.S.N. degree from

Eastern Michigan University. A registered nurse who has special-ized in burn care, she has worked in the field of risk management since 1986 and is certified as a health care risk management pro-fessional by the American Hospital Association. She has twice served as president of the Michigan Society of Healthcare Risk Man-agement (1994–95 and 1995–96) and is a member of the Amer-ican Society for Healthcare Risk Management. She is presently risk management consultant for health care at the University of Michigan.

Michael D. Fetters is a family physician and assistant professor in the Department of Family Medicine at the University of Michigan-Ann Arbor. His research in medical errors focuses on the primary care setting, and he is coauthor of the *Journal of Family Practice* ar-ticle "Adverse Events in Primary Care Identified from a Risk Man-agement Database." Fluent in Japanese as well as English, Fetters directs the University of Michigan Japanese Family Health Program, an initiative that seeks to provide comprehensive, linguistically and culturally sensitive care to the Japanese-speaking population of southeast Michigan (see www.med.umich.edu/jfhp for program information). He received his M.D. degree from the Ohio State University College of Medicine-Columbus, and completed family practice residency training at the University of North Carolina-Chapel Hill, where he also served as chief resident. During his Robert Wood Johnson Clinical Scholars Fellowship training at the University of North Carolina, he earned an M.P.H. degree from the School of Public Health Department of Epidemiology. He has also completed an M.A. degree with a concentration in anthropology and philosophy in the Inter-Disciplinary Program for Health and Humanities at Michigan State University.

Anne-Claire I. France is currently the director of the Center for Healthcare Improvement, the applied health services research arm of the Memorial Hermann Healthcare System in Houston, where patient safety is a priority. Her responsibilities include the organization's patient safety strategic plan, systems analysis for proactive error prevention, and cultural issues affecting patient safety. She also serves as the care transformation officer for implementation of a clinical information system derived from electronic medical records. She spearheads clinical practice improvement projects at Memorial Hermann; is president of Houston Health Innovations, LLC, which specializes in patient safety; and serves as vice chair of the Texas Forum on Health Safety. In addition, France teaches courses in applied health services research to health care administration graduate students. She received her Ph.D. degree in experimental psychology from Vanderbilt University and completed a postdoctoral research fellowship at the University of Texas Health Science Center Houston School of Medicine.

Robert L. Helmreich is professor of psychology at The University of Texas at Austin and director of the University of Texas Human Factors Research Project, which investigates human performance and threat and error management in aviation and medicine. Helmreich received the Flight Safety Foundation Distinguished Service Award in 1994 and is a member of the foundation's Icarus Committee. He is also a fellow of the Royal Aeronautical Society, the American Psychological Association, and the American Psychological Society. His research has been supported by the National Science Foundation, NASA, the Agency for Healthcare Research and Quality, and the Daimler-Benz Foundation. He is the author of more than two hundred publications, including *Culture at Work in Aviation and Medicine: National, Organizational, and Professional Influences* (with Ashleigh Merritt, 1998). He received his B.S., M.S., and Ph.D. degrees from Yale University.

Joanne V. Hickey is professor of clinical nursing at the University of Texas Health Science Center Houston. She is division head of Acute and Critical Care and director of the Acute Care Nurse Practitioner (ACNP) and Critical Care Clinical Nurse specialists programs, teaching in both these programs and the doctoral program.

An ACNP and APRN (advanced practice registered nurse) whose practice is focused on neuroscience patient populations, she is author of *The Clinical Practice of Neurological and Neurosurgical Nursing* (5th ed.) and senior editor of *Advanced Practice Nursing: Changing Roles and Clinical Applications*, now in its second edition. Hickey holds a Ph.D. degree, and her research is focused on blood pressure and heart rate variability in stroke patients and outcomes of neuroscience patients. She is a fellow in the American Academy of Nursing and the American College of Critical Care Medicine and chairperson of the Commission on Certification of the American Nurses Credentialing Center.

Susan D. Horn earned a B.A. degree in mathematics at Cornell University and a Ph.D. degree in statistics at Stanford University. She is senior scientist for the Institute for Clinical Outcomes Research (ICOR) and vice president of research for International Severity Information Systems, Inc. (ISIS), both located in Salt Lake City. In addition, she is a research professor in the Department of Medical Informatics at the University of Utah School of Medicine. Severity of illness measures developed by Horn and her colleagues were the basis for the Comprehensive Severity Index (CSI). Using CSI software, Horn has conducted clinical practice improvement (CPI) projects in a variety of areas. A frequent speaker on severity of illness and CPI methods used to determine best medical practice, Horn has authored over 130 publications and is coeditor of *Clinical Practice Improvement: A New Technology for Developing Cost Effective, Quality Health Care* (with David S. P. Hopkins, 1994) and editor of *Clinical Practice Improvement Methodology: Implementation and Evaluation* (1997).

Beverly Jones is vice president, patient care services and chief nursing officer, Henry Ford Health System, with leadership responsibility for nursing and other patient care services. She serves on the Henry Ford Hospital executive board, executive committee, and medical executive committee and is a member of the Henry Ford Health System and Henry Ford Hospital executive leadership teams. Jones came to the Henry Ford Health System from the University of Michigan Health System, where she served as chief of nursing and associate hospital director. She also served as associate dean in the University of Michigan School of Nursing. She holds a B.S.N. degree from Madonna College and an M.P.H. degree from the University of Michigan. A registered nurse, she is currently pursing a doctoral degree in nursing at Wayne State University. She is a fellow of the American Academy of Nursing and a member of the American Nurses Association and the American Organization of Nurse Executives.

Michael L. Millenson is Mervin Shalowitz, M.D., Visiting Scholar, Health Industry Management Program, Kellogg School of Management, Northwestern University, and a nationally recognized expert in health care quality, patient safety, and e-health. His book *Demanding Medical Excellence: Doctors and Accountability in the Information Age* (1997), funded by an Investigator Award in Health Policy Research from the Robert Wood Johnson Foundation, was the first examination of quality-of-care issues for a general audience. From 1996 to 2001, Millenson was a principal with William M. Mercer, Inc. Before that, as a long-time reporter for the *Chicago Tribune*, he was nominated for a Pulitzer Prize three times. Millenson's articles have appeared in such publications as *The Washington Monthly*, *Health Affairs*, and the *Journal of Health Politics, Policy and Law*. He has testified before Congress and the Institute of Medicine and is regularly quoted by the news media. He holds a B.A. degree from Washington University in St. Louis, where he was a member of the Economics Honor Society.

Ann P. Munro received a B.A. degree in political science from Wellesley College and an M.A. degree in public law and government-African studies from Columbia University before beginning her career in health care risk management with an M.P.H. degree from the University of Michigan. In addition to serving for twenty years in that university's Office of Medical Center Risk Management, she has been a long-time member in the Michigan Society of Healthcare Risk Management, holding the presidency in 1984–85, and an active participant in the American Society for Healthcare Risk Management, especially its risk identification and risk prevention activities related to university hospitals. She also played a central role in the Chicago-based University Hospitals Consortium risk management section. Her 1997 retirement from active employment as manager of the Office of Medical Center Risk Management also ended a long tenure on the University of Michigan Medical Center institutional review board.

Gilbert S. Omenn is executive vice president for medical affairs at the University of Michigan-Ann Arbor, CEO of the University of Michigan Health System, and professor in the Departments of Internal Medicine, Human Genetics, and Public Health. He was formerly dean of the School of Public Health and professor of medicine and environmental health at the University of Washington-Seattle. His research interests include chemoprevention of cancers, genetic predispositions to environmental and occupational health hazards, health promotion for older adults, science-based risk analysis, and health policy. The author of more than three hundred research papers and scientific reviews and author or editor of seventeen books, Omenn is a member of the Institute of Medicine and a fellow of the American College of Physicians, and he serves on the board of directors of Rohm & Haas and Amgen. He chaired the federal Commission on Risk Assessment and Risk Management (the Omenn Commission) and the National Academy of Sciences/National Research Council/Institute of Medicine Committee on Science, Engineering and Public Policy. Omenn holds a B.A. degree from Princeton University, an M.D. degree magna cum laude from Harvard Medical School, and a Ph.D. degree in genetics from the University of Washington.

Paul R. Schulman is Robert and Ann Wert Professor of Government at Mills College in Oakland, California, and he has also taught at the University of Tennessee, University of California-Berkeley, and Brown University in the general area of science, technology, and public policy making. His recent research and writing has focused on the special challenges organizations face in managing hazardous technologies safely and reliably. In this connection, he has examined nuclear power plants, air traffic control, electrical grid reliability, and most recently, medical organizations. Among his publications are *Modelling the Growth of Federal Agencies and Programs* and *Large-Scale Policy-Making*. He earned a B.A. degree from Tulane University and M.A. and Ph.D. degrees from The Johns Hopkins University.

David M. Studdert is assistant professor of law and public health at the Harvard School of Public Health, where he teaches courses in health law and medical ethics. His research focuses on legal and regulatory issues in the health care sector, and he is currently involved in a series of projects investigating medical injury, coverage appeals in managed care organizations, and workplace discrimination. Previously, he worked as a policy analyst at RAND and as an adviser to the minister for health in Australia and practiced commercial litigation. Studdert holds an L.L.B. degree and an Sc.D. degree in public health and health policy.

Eric J. Thomas is assistant professor of medicine at the University of Texas Houston Medical School. He attended the University of Texas (UT) at Austin and received his M.D. degree from the University of Texas Southwestern Medical School. He then received a M.P.H. degree from Harvard University and joined the Harvard Medical School faculty before joining the UT Houston Medical School in 1998. He also serves as a general internist at Memorial Hermann Hospital. Since 1992, he has conducted research on patient safety, and his work was heavily cited in the Institute of Medicine landmark report on medical error. For three years he has

collaborated closely with Robert Helmreich to translate safety practices from aviation to health care. Thomas's research has been supported by the Robert Wood Johnson Foundation and the U.S.
Agency for Healthcare Research and Quality.

Derek van Amerongen serves as vice president and chief medical
officer for Humana/ChoiceCare in Cincinnati, overseeing medical
management and strategy for one of the nation's most innovative
and prestigious health plans. He is also on the faculty of Xavier
University's School of Health Administration. Previously, he was
national medical director for Anthem Blue Cross and Blue Shield,
responsible for working with national accounts as well as creating
and directing that company's women's health initiative, and a faculty member in The Johns Hopkins School of Medicine Department of Gynecology and Obstetrics. Van Amerongen has written
and presented extensively on managed care and health policy. His
first book, *Networks and the Future of Medical Practice*, won the 1998
Robert A. Henry Literary Award of the American College of Physician Executives. He received his B.S. degree from Princeton University, his M.S. degree in medical administration from the
University of Wisconsin, and his M.D. degree from Rush Medical
College. He performed his residency in obstetrics and gynecology
at the University of Chicago and is board certified in that specialty.

Karl E. Weick is Rensis Likert Distinguished University Professor of
Organizational Behavior and Psychology and Professor of Psychology at the University of Michigan. He has also held faculty positions at the University of Texas, Cornell University, University of
Minnesota, and Purdue University. Weick earned his Ph.D. degree
in social and organizational psychology from Ohio State University, and is a former editor of the *Administrative Science Quarterly*
(1977 to 1985), former associate editor of the journal *Organizational
Behavior and Human Performance*, and current topic editor (human
factors) at the journal *Wildfire*. His research interests include col-

lective sensemaking under pressure, medical errors, handoffs and transitions in dynamic events, high reliability performance, improvisation, and continuous change. His current writing is distributed across a variety of projects that include a reanalysis of the Dude wildland fire in 1990 in which six firefighters perished; a discussion of organizational scholars' mechanisms for intellectual renewal; a review of leadership lessons learned from wildland fire tragedies; and a generalization of research findings on high reliability organizations to the larger issue of high-performing organizations; and investigation of distributed sensemaking in the West Nile and hantavirus outbreaks.

Medical Error

Part One

Setting the Stage

Although physicians have been worrying about and studying *adverse events* for as long as the profession of medicine has existed, systematic, large-scale studies are recent phenomena. The single most comprehensive such effort is the Harvard Medical Practice Study of adverse events in a random sample of State of New York hospitals, released in 1990.

Ten years later, a special committee of the Institute of Medicine published *To Err Is Human*, an important exploration of medical error. This report relied heavily on the findings of the Harvard Medical Practice Study. It also included important work from other disciplines such as human factors engineering and high reliability organization theory, which explore the influence of organizational conditions and systems elements on human error.

Part One of this book provides a comprehensive review of the original Harvard Medical Practice Study in Chapter One, and looks at ways that study may have been misinterpreted. This chapter also summarizes findings from more recent research conducted by some of the original HMPS investigators. It highlights the scale and importance of the problem. It also points out the weaknesses inherent in conducting studies of this sort. It explores the complications and contortions produced by our country's reliance on the tort system for settling malpractice disputes. Perhaps the most serious impact of that reliance is the chilling effect malpractice threats have on medical error reporting.

By discussing how the HMPS started the current national discussion of medical error and where we have come since its publication, Part One offers a fitting beginning for this book's exploration of what we know and what we do.

1

What Have We Learned Since the Harvard Medical Practice Study?

David M. Studdert, Troyen A. Brennan, and Eric J. Thomas

Interest in the study of medical injury gained momentum through the 1990s, culminating in the Institute of Medicine's report *To Err Is Human* (Kohn, Corrigan, & Donaldson, 2000). The report brought unprecedented attention to the field among researchers and the general public — publicity that will no doubt provide the impetus for numerous studies of error and injury in the years ahead. New research in this area is welcome, both because of the gravity of the problem and our currently limited knowledge.

A significant contribution to what we do currently know about medical mistakes and malpractice litigation comes from a series of studies of iatrogenic injury, its economic consequences, and the resolution of associated claims. Pioneering work was undertaken in California in the late 1970s and early 1980s. Responding to a perceived crisis in malpractice litigation in the mid-1970s, the California Medical Association and the California Hospital Association

---

Revised from David M. Studdert, Troyen A. Brennan, and Eric J. Thomas, *Beyond Dead Reckoning: Measures of Medical Injury Burden, Malpractice Litigation, and Alternative Compensation Models from Utah and Colorado*, Indiana Law Review, 2000, 33, 1643. Copyright 2000, The Trustees of Indiana University. Reproduced with permission from the *Indiana Law Review*.

jointly commissioned the Medical Insurance Feasibility Study (MIFS)—an investigation of medical records designed to measure rates of injury in hospitalized patients (California Medical Association & California Hospital Association, 1977; see also Mills, 1978). A team of medico-legal experts, led by Don Harper Mills, reviewed nearly 21,000 records in twenty-three hospitals across the state and found 970 incidents of disability caused by health care management. Because the hospitals were carefully selected to be representative of hospitals statewide in terms of size, ownership, teaching status, and region, the findings implied that approximately 4.6 percent of Californians hospitalized in the mid-1970s (roughly one in twenty) suffered some sort of iatrogenic injury. One in every one hundred inpatients suffered an injury that gave rise to permanent or grave disability.

In the midst of a second surge in malpractice claims in the mid 1980s, a group of Harvard investigators undertook a similar evaluation of malpractice litigation in New York State (Harvard Medical Practice Study, 1990). The objective of the Harvard Medical Practice Study (HMPS) was to answer three questions: (1) How frequently do medical injuries occur in hospitals, particularly the subset of injuries attributable to negligent care? (2) What portion of those injuries gives rise to litigation, and conversely, how much litigation proceeds in the absence of such injuries? and (3) What are the economic consequences of medical injuries?

This chapter revisits the results of the HMPS in light of new information about medical injury and malpractice litigation. In particular we report findings from a recently completed set of investigations in Utah and Colorado, which replicated many of the HMPS methods. The chapter begins by reviewing the HMPS and describing several important changes to the health care system that made repetition of this kind of large-scale study of iatrogenic injury worthwhile. Next we outline results from each of the four main areas of analysis comprised by the Utah-Colorado Medical Practice Study (UCMPS): incidence of medical injury, malpractice claiming behavior, the economic consequences of medical injury, and the feasibility of alternative approaches to compensation. In conclusion we summarize our findings and discuss their implications for health care policy.

The Harvard Medical Practice Study and Its Findings

Led by Howard Hiatt, M.D., the former dean of the Harvard School of Public Health, the HMPS investigators quickly recognized that the dual tasks of charting the epidemiology of medical injury and malpractice claims would require a medico-legal data collection effort on an unprecedented scale. Hiatt secured a significant funding commitment from the New York Department of Health and from the Robert Wood Johnson Foundation. After three years of design work, the investigators commenced data collection in New York.

HMPS investigators assembled a representative sample of fifty-two hospitals from among the more than three hundred acute care facilities in New York, and randomly sampled medical records for the year 1984 from those hospitals (for a full description of the HMPS sampling methodology, see Harvard Medical Practice Study, 1990, chap. 4.). The study sample was weighted to allow statistical transformation of results from this selection of institutions and records into statewide estimates. Teams of physicians and nurses then reviewed each record, looking for evidence of *adverse events*—defined as injuries caused by medical practice, as opposed to a disease process, that either prolonged the patient's hospital stay or resulted in disability at the time of discharge. When an adverse event was detected, the chart review protocol directed the physician reviewers to judge whether it had been caused by negligence. Negligence was defined, in accordance with standard tort criteria, as actual injuries proximately resulting from a treating physician's failure to meet the standard of care expected in his or her practice community (Prosser, Keeton, & Dobbs, 1984, § 30, pp. 164–165).

While record review proceeded, the investigators contacted more than twenty insurance companies underwriting malpractice risk in New York for injury year 1984. Unfortunately, by the time this process began in 1990, the effects of a second tort crisis in the mid-1980s had been felt. Many insurers had gone into state receivership, having failed as a result of unanticipated increases in expenditures on litigation and settlements. This made the task of identifying claims quite arduous. Nonetheless, investigators successfully created a database of nearly 68,000 malpractice claims filed between 1984 and 1989. Patients were then linked to claimants using software programs designed to maximize the identification of name matches. In this way, investigators were able to identify which patients whose medical records were examined in the chart review were subsequently involved in litigation.

Finally, a survey of individuals who had suffered adverse events gathered information on the economic consequences of the injuries. This survey occurred more than four years after the injury itself to allow investigators to make a reasonable assessment of the repercussions of the injury. Unfortunately, respondents' ability to recall actual costs appeared to be significantly impaired by the time elapsed. The site team applied unit cost estimates to information obtained in the surveys to assess overall costs of injury (Johnson et al., 1992).

The results of the HMPS have been widely reported (for a summary of articles published through 1993, see Weiler et al., 1993, pp. 155–175). The investigators detected a slightly lower rate of adverse events than had been found in MIFS. Approximately 3.7 percent of patients hospitalized in New York in 1984 were estimated to have suffered a medical injury associated with their stay (Brennan et al., 1991). Just over one-quarter of those injuries were due to negligence. When these figures were *up-weighted* to account for all hospital discharges in the state, they indicated that 100,000 New Yorkers suffered medical injuries in 1984, 13,000 of which resulted in death. Negligence gave rise to approximately 20,000 disabling injuries and 7,000 deaths.

These alarming statistics have become the chief legacy of the HMPS. For the first time, the burden of morbidity and mortality from medical injuries was widely publicized. This attention, in turn, helped to spawn interest in error measurement and prevention — one of the most vibrant fields of inquiry in health services research today (Leape, 1994, 1998). Efforts to understand medical error, however, remain largely contained within a frame of analysis concerned with quality of clinical care. Commentators and researchers involved in the study of error — many of them clinicians — typically view the law's role with disdain and pay it little attention. Few have explored legal means for deterring accidents (Liang, 1999).

The patient safety movement's orientation away from scrutiny of the legal system is problematic, given the solid evidence from the HMPS that the tort system has been failing in both its compensation and deterrence functions. In total, approximately 3,600 malpractice claims relating to injury year 1984 were made in New York (Localio et al., 1991). A comparison to the 27,000 negligent adverse events arising in that year produces a negligence-to-claims ratio of 7.5 to 1 — not much smaller than the ratio identified by Danzon (1985) using data from the MIFS a decade earlier. Even when the injury sample is narrowed to a subset of more monetarily valuable tort claims — those involving serious injury to patients less than seventy years old — a negligence-to-claims ratio of 5 to 2 persists (Weiler et al., 1993, p. 71).

But the HMPS analysis of litigation went a step further than the MIFS analysis had by matching specific claims to specific injuries. This exercise shed new light on the dimensions of the disconnection between claims and injuries: not only did few documented instances of negligent injury give rise to claims, the majority of claims that were initiated did not appear to be grounded in identifiable instances of negligence. Investigators estimated that, among the 3,600 claims in New York relating to injury suffered in 1984, more than one-half arose from instances in which there was neither negligence nor any identifiable injury, and one-third arose from instances of injury but no negligence; only one-sixth corresponded to "true" negligent incidents (Localio et al., 1991).

We have previously described this paradoxical relationship as both lopsided and mismatched (Studdert et al., 2000). Paul Weiler draws an analogy to a traffic officer ticketing random drivers, a process that penalizes some violaters, but also some nonviolaters, and allows many violaters to pass (Weiler et al., 1993, p. 75).[1] This dysfunctional situation clearly implies that compensation and deterrence objectives are not fully realized by malpractice law. In fact the only clear evidence of a relationship between malpractice claiming and actual behavioral responses found in the HMPS was at the level of the hospital, and here the important signal was the overall number of medical injuries, not the number of medical injuries actually due to negligence (Brennan, 1998). This finding intimated that institutions may be best positioned to channel the liability threat and experience toward injury-reduction strategies, an argument made persuasively by several legal commentators (see Abraham & Weiler, 1994; Sage, Hastings, & Berenson, 1994) and one that resonates with contemporary organizational theories of safety. Overall, HMPS investigators did not interpret their findings about the dynamics of litigation as supporting ongoing reliance on individually targeted tort litigation to ensure patient safety (Weiler et al., 1993, pp. 139–149).

The Need for Validation

Given such clear-cut findings about the incidence of medical injury and the dynamics of malpractice litigation, why should the HMPS require validation? The most obvious reasons stem from a couple of significant market transitions in the United States. Perhaps most important, managed care has emerged as a major force in U.S. medicine. The penetration of managed care in New York in 1984 was minimal. Managed care's rapid rise began in the late 1980s, not only in New York but also in many other regions of the country, and within several years managed care had taken root as a new way of life in the practice of medicine. The other market shift concerns proprietary medicine. New York had no for-profit sector of hospital care in 1984. By the early 1990s, for-profit institutions were well established in many markets around the United States, including those in New York. Managed care, for-profit medicine, and the points of intersection between these two phenomena have largely transformed the health care industry that existed before 1990. It is unclear what effect these changes are likely to have on the rate and types of medical injuries, although the industry's greater emphasis on financial considerations has undoubtedly elevated concerns about errors of omission (as opposed to commission).

Issues of generalizability aside, a series of recurring questions has arisen about aspects of the HMPS itself. First, with regard to identification of medical injuries, a number of critics have pointed out that the reliability of judgments about injury and negligence is less than stellar (see, for example, Anderson, 1996; Brennan, Localio, & Laird, 1989; Localio et al., 1996). Second, questions have persisted about the extent of the gap identified between numbers of malpractice claims and of medical injuries in the HMPS; most other studies of malpractice claims suggest a smaller mismatch between claims and negligence (see Taragin, Willet, Wilczek, Trout, & Carson, 1992; White, 1994). Third, the task of collecting data on malpractice claims in New York proved particularly challenging due to the volatile malpractice environment that existed in 1984. Fourth, HMPS investigators did not have the tools to estimate the costs of different compensation models or to compare these costs to those of the tort system; consequently, assessments of the economic feasibility of alternative schemes, such as *no-fault* compensation, were crude.

En masse, this set of defects and unanswered questions is very serious. Before policymakers could reasonably be expected to rely on the HMPS findings, we believed it was necessary to validate that study. In preparing to bring the medical injury statistics up to date, we sought states that differed markedly from New York, both regionally and in their demographic mix. Another important criterion was the existence of a mature health care industry, including a managed care and for-profit hospital presence. To simplify and improve the study of malpractice litigation, we also hoped to find states with relatively stable, monopolistic indemnity insurance markets.

The Utah-Colorado Medical Practice Study

In 1995, the Robert Wood Johnson Foundation provided us with a grant to undertake a study similar to the HMPS in Utah and Colorado. We worked closely with the legislatures and the dominant physician malpractice insurers in these two states. Collaborators provided us with an unprecedented level of access to hospital data systems and malpractice claims. In collecting and analyzing these data, we redeployed the basic methods of the HMPS, making several design changes and running repairs in places where we thought significant deficiencies existed. The lead results of the UCMPS were recently reported in the medical literature (see Thomas et al., 1999, 2000a; Studdert et al., 2000).

The Health Burden of Medical Injury

Our validation goals demanded that the pool of injuries detected in the mountain states be directly comparable with that from New York. As we have noted, however, the reliability of record reviewers' judgments—both adverse event and negligence determinations—was a major focus of the methodological critiques that followed release of the New York findings. Drawing on knowledge gained from work done in the interim on *inter-rater reliability* and from ongoing analyses of the New York experience, we made several modifications to the review process. Most notably, we revamped reviewer-training practices and instituted a series of quality checks on physician reviewers' judgments.

From thirteen representative hospitals in Utah and fifteen in Colorado, we completed reviews of 4,943 (98.9 percent) of 5,000 sampled records in Utah and 9,757 (97.6 percent) of 10,000 records in Colorado. Physician reviewers identified a total of 169 adverse events in Utah and 418 adverse events in Colorado. When these totals are up-weighted to the state populations, they yield estimates of 5,614 adverse events among hospitalized patients in Utah in 1992, and 11,578 in Colorado. We estimated an adverse event rate of 2.9 percent in both states, a remarkable similarity considering that medical records were reviewed by completely different teams of physicians in each state. In Utah 32.6 percent of the adverse events were judged due to negligence; in Colorado the proportion was 27.5 percent.

To analyze types of adverse events, we pooled the results. As Table 1.1 illustrates, the most prevalent injury type was adverse events connected to surgery, accounting for approximately half (44.9 percent) of adverse events across both states (for a detailed analysis of the surgical adverse events identified in the UCMPS, see Gawande, Thomas, Zinner, & Brennan, 1999). Nearly one-third of these were the result of technical complications in the operation. Only 16.9 percent of surgical adverse events involved negligence. Approximately the same proportion resulted in permanent disability.

Drug-related adverse events were the next most prevalent group. They accounted for more than one-third of the balance of the injuries. The four most common classes of drugs involved were antibiotics (24.9 percent), cardiovascular agents (17.4 percent), analgesics (8.9 percent), and anticoagulants (8.6 percent). Strikingly, more than one-third of all drug-related adverse events detected were due to negligence. The mistakes included prescription of the wrong drug (20.9 percent), prescription of the wrong dose (7.9 percent), and prescription of a drug to a patient with a known allergy to that drug (5.7 percent).[2]

Table 1.1. Types of Adverse Events.

Type	Adverse Events	%[a]	% of Adverse Events with Negligence
Operative	7,715	44.9	16.9
Technical	2,309	29.9	23.6
Bleeding	1,319	17.1	9.8
Wound infection	877	11.4	20.8
Nonwound infection	775	10.0	7.5
Drug-related	3,325	19.3	35.1
Antibiotic	828	24.9	6.8
Cardiovascular agent	579	17.4	38.9
Analgesic	297	8.9	33.3
Anticoagulant	286	8.6	25.1
Medical procedure	2,315	13.5	15.3
Incorrect or delayed diagnosis	1,181	6.9	93.8
Incorrect or delayed therapy	736	4.3	56.8
Postpartum	620	3.6	25.5
Neonatal	532	3.1	25.3
Anesthesia-related	226	1.3	32.7
Falls	220	1.3	65.8
Fracture-related	66	0.4	0
Other	256	1.5	59.9
Total	17,192		

[a] Percentages shown for the subtypes of operative and drug-related adverse events represent proportions of the total number of adverse events in the relevant category (that is, 7,715 and 3,325, respectively).

Compared to the findings from New York, iatrogenic death was a relatively rare occurrence in the mountain states. Only 6.6 percent of adverse events resulted in death, although the death rate was slightly higher (8.8 percent) among negligent adverse events. In total, 439 patients hospitalized in Utah and Colorado in 1992 died due to negligent care; another 160 victims of negligence suffered grave or major disability.

These mortality statistics confirm the existence of an epidemic of potentially preventable iatrogenic death in the United States. However, they present a considerably less bleak picture than emerged from New York eight years earlier. When extrapolated to the U.S. population, iatrogenic deaths detected in the HMPS suggested nearly 200,000 deaths a year were due to adverse events, whereas the UCMPS suggests approximately 65,000 deaths. The difference widens for negligent adverse events: 120,000 negligent deaths nationwide versus somewhat fewer than 25,000, extrapolating from the HMPS and the UCMPS rates respectively. This five-fold difference in deaths due to negligent care is particularly striking.

There are several explanations for it. First, by the time we initiated the UCMPS, we had become aware of a growing literature suggesting that severity of injury tended to inappropriately color judgments about quality of care (see, for example, Hayward, Bernard, Rosevear, Anderson, & McMahon, 1993). Therefore, during reviewer training, we dealt specifically with the need to differentiate injury severity from the judgment of causation or negligence. Second, the standard of medical care may simply have been better in Colorado and Utah in 1992 than in New York in 1984. Third, we cannot, of course, rule out the possibility that limitations in the methods we used, principally chart review, at least partly explain disparities between the two studies (for a recent critique of the questionable role of reviewer consensus, see Hofer, Berstein, De Monner, & Hayward, 2000).

But despite the differences noted, the story that emerges from comparison of the HMPS and UCMPS results is chiefly one of tremendous similarity. Beginning with the overall adverse event rate itself, there is no statistically significant difference between the proportions of hospital discharges involving patients who have experienced adverse events. Cross-study analyses of a variety of other measures show that the UCMPS findings essentially reinforce those from the HMPS. For example, the proportion of operative adverse events is stable between studies. Slightly more than one-half of all negligent adverse events in both studies occurred in the emergency department, and a very high proportion of all adverse events attributed to emergency physicians were judged to be due to negligence (70.4 percent in New York and 52.6 percent in Utah and Colorado). Together, the studies provide overwhelming evidence that the burden of iatrogenic injury is large, enduring, and an innate feature of hospital care in the United States.

Two other studies since the HMPS have yielded contrasting results and warrant mention. In August 1995, to much public clamor, the Australian government announced results from the Quality in Australian Health Care Study (QAHCS). Ross Wilson and colleagues (1995) estimated that 16.6 percent of admissions to Australian hospitals were associated with adverse events, 51 percent of which were considered preventable.[3] Having consulted with QAHCS investigators throughout their study, we were surprised by these results because the Australians also drew a sample from 1992, identical in size to the UCMPS sample, and then modeled their methods, as we had, on those developed during the HMPS. Yet they detected nearly six times more adverse events than the UCMPS did. A closer analysis of the respective study methods and samples showed that several relatively straightforward adjustments were necessary to allow direct comparability (Thomas et al., 2000b). However, such adjustments still reduced the disparity only to a fourfold difference.

The UCMPS results are also quite different from those obtained in a 1997 study by Lori Andrews and colleagues (1997) in Illinois. Using ethnographic measurement techniques to track adverse events occurring in "real time," they found a rate of 17.7 percent in one university teaching hospital. However, fairly major differences between the Andrews study and the UCMPS in sampling and other aspects of the methodologies limit the studies' comparability.[4]

The Relationship Between Malpractice Claims and Medical Injuries

An important component of the UCMPS, like the HMPS before it, was to link the medical injuries identified in record review to malpractice claims. The task was less onerous than had been the case in New York, thanks to a more stable claims environment in the mountain states, more detailed and readily accessible claims files, and the existence of several dominant indemnity insurers. All the leading insurers contributed claims data. We then used computer-matching techniques to identify patients from the medical record review who filed malpractice claims during or after 1992.

We identified eighteen claims arising from records we had reviewed, eight in Utah and ten in Colorado. The low number of matches was expected, given the relatively small sample size of both medical records and claims in the UCMPS. Nonetheless, we were still able to link the claims information with chart review findings and sketch an empirical picture of the relationship between medical injuries and malpractice litigation. Table 1.2 summarizes this relationship and compares the UCMPS findings to those from New York and California. The data tell quite a consistent story about the claims-negligence dynamic.

Markedly different litigation environments prevailed in the four states at the time of each study (see row 1). California and New York were experiencing frenetic claims activity, whereas the situation in Utah and Colorado was relatively calm at the time of our medico-legal measurements. The high litigation rates on the East and West coasts are no doubt partly attributable to the medical malpractice "crises" that unfolded in the mid-1970s and mid-1980s. However, California and New York are distinctive in other ways that could affect claims, incidence of negligence, and claims-negligence dynamics: both are heavily populated, are among the states with the highest lawyer-to-population ratios, and are renowned for having consistently high rates of malpractice litigation.

Table 1.2. Relationship Between Negligent Adverse Events and Claims.

Relationship	Utah 1992	Colorado 1992	New York 1984	California 1976
Claims per 100 physicians per year	7.1	7.3	14.0	17.4
Negligent adverse event rate (per 100 discharges)	0.90	0.80	1.00	0.79
Ratio of negligent adverse events to claims	5.1	6.7	7.6	10.0
Probability claim follows negligent adverse event	2.5%		1.5%	—

Row 2 of Table 1.2 restates findings from the chart reviews: it illustrates that volume of litigation has no significant bearing on the incidence of malpractice. Nor do litigation rates appear to affect accuracy of claiming, as shown in row 4. However, fewer claims combined with steady negligence rates must mean that the "malpractice gap" narrows. Row 3 shows that the degree to which instances of substandard care outstrip claims that allege such care was less in Utah (ratio of 5.1. to 1) and Colorado (ratio of 6.7 to 1) than it was in the high litigation states of New York (ratio of 7.6 to 1) and California (ratio of 10.0 to 1). Taken together, the data in Table 1.2 suggest that the dysfunctional characteristics of the medical malpractice system —most notably, its *adequacy* and its *accuracy*—when viewed through an epidemiological lens, have a resilience over time and across jurisdictions.

An important caveat is in order at this point. Regardless of the similarity between the methods that generated these comparative data, any conclusions about intertemporal and cross-regional trends must be tempered by an acknowledgment that the data are not longitudinal. Because we have no evidence that the disconnection observed between negligent injury and claiming behavior existed in the mountain states in earlier periods, we are unable to infer that it is insensitive to overall rates of claims and stable across time and regions of the country. However, our findings certainly lend plausibility to the argument that the findings from Utah, Colorado, New York, and California are a reasonable reflection of the situation in other states.

The final analysis in the malpractice component of the UCMPS was focused on the significant population of patients—more than 97 percent of those who suffered negligent adverse events in our study—who experience malpractice but never file claims seeking compensation. To profile this group, we compared UCMPS information on 157 patients from Colorado who were found to have suffered negligence but had not sued with information on individuals who had sued for injuries allegedly suffered in 1992. (Information on the latter group was obtained directly from insurers.)

Our results are shown in Table 1.3. Predictably, people who did not claim despite having suffered negligence were more likely to have suffered minor injury. Nonclaimants were also much more likely to be Medicare recipients, Medicaid recipients, seventy-five years old or older, and low-income earners. These findings support and elaborate those of Burstin, Johnson, Lipsitz, and Brennan (1993) from the HMPS.

How can the strong association between the sociodemographic factors we identified and underclaiming be explained? Financial incentives provide one explanation. Economic theories of tort law suggest that individuals who are poor or who do not earn income, whether or not they are poor, will be less likely to sue. Malpractice litigation is rarely initiated without attorney involvement, hence a prospective litigant's ability to claim typically hinges on an attorney's willingness to take on the case. Because the financial return accruing to plaintiffs' attorneys in tort cases is generally linked to the size of the award through contingency fees, and lost income typically forms a significant component of malpractice awards, these lawyers would tend to maximize their own income by choosing to act for clients with ongoing sources of income. (Indeed, the

Table 1.3. Multivariate Odds of Failure to Claim Despite Negligence, by Sociodemographic Characteristics (Colorado, incident year 1992).

Characteristics	Odds Ratio	95% Confidence Interval
	Nonclaimants compared to all claimants *(n = 109 and 256, respectively)*	
Female	1.4	0.8–2.6
Patient age[a]		
< 18	1.0	0.3–3.3
45 to 64	1.7	0.8–3.6
65 to 74	2.2	0.6–7.3
≥ 75	7.0	1.7–29.6*
Payer[b]		
Medicare	3.5	1.3–9.6*
Medicaid	3.6	1.4–9.0*
Uninsured	2.0	0.7–5.8
Income[c]		
Poor	2.0	0.8–5.3
Low income	2.0	0.9–4.2**
High income	0.8	0.3–1.8
Disability[d]		
Minor	6.3	2.7–14.9*
Significant	1.7	0.8–3.9

[a] Reference group was patients aged 18 to 44 years. [b] Reference group was privately insured. [c] Reference group was middle income. [d] Reference group was major disability.

$* P < 0.05.$ $** P < 0.1.$

costs of bringing a claim may simply exceed the damages recoverable.) The elderly and the poor are particularly unlikely to generate income. Moreover, any income they do generate is less likely to be "lost" owing to a decline in physical capacity occasioned by negligent injury. In addition, the size of any award to elderly patients will usually be constrained by their shorter life expectancy.

Other factors that we did not account for in our statistical analysis, such as regulatory barriers (see Legal Services Corporation Act,

1999; McNulty, 1989) and level of education, may also play a role in defining the nonclaimant group. But whatever the true underlying cause of patients' failure to claim despite having suffered negligence, the critique leveled at the efficacy of the current malpractice system is the same: factors other than individual merit appear to play a strong role in determining who uses the malpractice system and who receives compensation from it. These concerns should be understood in the context of our more general findings that claims lag well behind the incidence of negligent injury, and the two are seldom connected in the current system.

Economic Burden of Medical Injury

Using information obtained in surveys of injured patients, HMPS investigators estimated that adverse events among patients hospitalized in New York in 1984 led to $3.8 billion in total health care costs (Johnson et al., 1992). This figure implied total national costs of slightly more than $50 billion in 1984. After carefully weighing a mix of considerations, including residual reservations about potential recall biases among HMPS patients, resource constraints, and the ethical complexities associated with recontacting patients with knowledge in hand about both injuries they had suffered and causes of those injuries, we chose to use experts' judgments of costs instead of patient surveys in the UCMPS. The specific methods used to estimate each of the key expenditure items—lost wages, lost household production, and health care costs—are described in detail elsewhere (Thomas et al., 1999).

We estimated that the economic consequences of the adverse events in Utah and Colorado in 1992 totaled $661.9 million. The subset of adverse events judged to have been preventable accounted for nearly one-half of this total, or $308.3 million. Postoperative complications and adverse drug events were the most expensive type of adverse events, with the former giving rise to $232.0 million in costs and the latter, $213.7 million.

Table 1.4 shows that the largest share of the total was accounted for by health care costs. More than $348 million was spent on treatment in response to adverse events suffered in hospitals in the two states in 1992. Surprisingly, one-half of these health care costs were attributable to nursing home care expenditures. Inpatient hospital costs absorbed the next largest portion (41 percent), followed by non-intensive care bed days (31 percent) and intensive care (10 percent). In total, the health care costs of adverse events in Utah and Colorado that accrued in outpatient settings, inclusive of nursing home costs, were nearly twice as large as the inpatient costs. This finding is all the more remarkable when one considers that the UCMPS focused on adverse events suffered in the inpatient setting.

When extrapolated to the thirty-three million discharges from U.S. hospitals in 1992, our estimates put the annual costs of adverse events nationwide at approximately $38 billion. This is smaller than, although not greatly dissimilar from, the $50 billion figure derived from patient interviews in the HMPS. Some of this difference is driven by the slightly higher adverse event rate detected in New York. When adjusted to 1996 dollars and recalculated with UCMPS adverse event rates, the New York data suggest annual costs of $147 per capita; the UCMPS estimates are $132 per capita. The proximity of the two estimates is noteworthy given the quite different methodological approaches used to derive them.

One lesson from our cost analyses concerns the importance of looking expansively at health care costs in estimating the effects of iatrogenic injury. Despite the fact that the UCMPS gathered data on inpatient injuries, we nonetheless found more than 60 percent of total health care costs arising outside the hospital. This suggests that other studies of adverse events that have focused exclusively on inpatient costs—for example, those undertaken in the field of drug-related adverse events (Bates et al., 1997; Classen, Pestotnik, Evans, Lloyd, & Burke, 1997)—are likely to have missed the full economic implications of the medical injuries they examined. Efforts to understand the implications of injuries in a broader range

Table 1.4. Adverse Event Costs in Utah and Colorado (in thousands, discounted to 1996 dollars).

	All Adverse Events (%)	Preventable Adverse Events (%)
Health care costs	348,081 (53)	59,245 (52)
Lost wages	160,946 (24)	63,309 (20)
Lost household production	152,862 (23)	85,828 (28)
Total	661,889 (100)	308,382 (100)

of health care settings have begun (Gandhi et al., 2000) and will add vital information to the knowledge base.

Our findings also provide some targets for improvement. The most costly areas appear to be adverse surgical events, adverse drug events, and adverse events due to incorrect diagnoses. Front-end expenditures devoted to preventing medical error in these areas could yield savings overall, although precise estimates of the cost trade-offs involved are desperately needed. Thus the next phase of research into the economic consequences of medical injury may well belong to cost-effectiveness analysts. But even without the benefit of such analyses, the economic research to date suggests that as a whole, U.S. hospitals are almost certainly underspending in their efforts to prevent adverse events. More than one-half of the adverse events we detected were judged preventable. If such prevention occurred, it could relieve the U.S. health care system of nearly $20 billion in health care costs, or 2 percent of present health care expenditures.

The Persistent Question: How to Improve Compensation for Medical Injuries?

Many commentators have suggested that alternative strategies for compensating medical injuries should be considered in the United States (see, for example, Havighurst & Tancredi, 1973; O'Connell, 1975; Saks, 1992; Sugarman, 1985). An administrative system, somewhat similar to current workers' compensation regimes, that does not make compensation contingent on proof that fault or negligence caused the injury in question, has long been heralded by some as the best candidate (Weiler, 1993). But concerns have been raised about a pure no-fault system, the principal one being that such a system would be inordinately expensive to operate in this country (Abramson, 1989–1990; Bovbjerg, 1993; Mashaw & Marmor, 1994; Saks, 1994; Sugarman, 1991).

Given the policy imperatives that motivated the UCMPS, a key study goal from the outset was to evaluate the economic feasibility of a practical, workable no-fault scheme. Building on work done by Marilynn Rosenthal, Randall Bovbjerg, and Lawrence Tancredi, we investigated design options. We were attracted to the Swedish Patient Injury Compensation Fund (see Rosenthal, 1987; Oldertz, 1998). Sweden has successfully operated this fund, an administrative compensation program, for the past two decades. The criteria used do not contemplate all adverse events as compensable injuries. Rather, they incorporate consideration of the *avoidability* of the injury — a notion we have previously described in detail (see Studdert et al., 1997). We hypothesized that a no-fault program designed around Swedish compensation criteria would demarcate a generous, yet manageable body of medical injuries as eligible for compensation. In terms of volume, the pool of injuries contemplated lies between all adverse events (that is, pure no-fault) and negligent adverse events (that is, the malpractice system).

We applied Swedish compensation criteria to the pool of injuries detected in the UCMPS. Table 1.5 shows that this exercise resulted in estimates of a total compensation budget, including projected administrative costs, that are significantly lower than the total injury costs obtained in our earlier analysis of the economic consequences of medical injury. Costs are further decreased if an eight-week disability (or *deductible*) period is added as a prerequisite to accessing compensation.[5] In Utah, the total for compensating the Swedish compensable events with an eight-week disability period was $76.8 million. In Colorado, the cost was almost exactly $100 million.

Table 1.6 examines the affordability of candidate no-fault schemes, comparing their estimated cost to the estimated cost of the current medical malpractice system in each state. According to our best estimates and those of our collaborators in Utah and Colorado, malpractice premiums paid in those states in 1996 totaled approximately $60 million and $100 million respectively. In Utah, one approach to compensation under consideration during the UCMPS proposed use of Swedish compensable events, a $100,000 cap on pain and suffering, a four-week disability period, exclusion of household production, and 66 percent wage replacement. The estimated cost of such a program, after addition of administrative and birth injury costs, would be $54.9 million (in 1992 dollars). In Colorado, the preferred model also involved use of Swedish compensable events, an eight-week disability period, full wage replacement, and exclusion of household production. Our calculations suggested total system costs of $102.4 million for Colorado.

Thus our cost estimates for the Swedish-style systems in Utah and Colorado compare favorably to the tort system: at $54.9 million, the Utah model would cost approximately the same as the tort system, whereas at $82 million, the Colorado model would be expected actually to reduce the costs of compensating medical injury by $18 million to $28 million annually. To keep these estimates in perspective, it is worth noting that in 1992, our study year, total personal health care expenditures were $3.8 billion in Utah and $9.4 billion in Colorado (see Levit et al., 1995, table 11).

Table 1.7 shows the *ratcheting* effects of removing household production and pain and suffering, items that some policymakers may believe are dispensable in a system of compensation. The table also shows how the number of beneficiaries shifts with the selection of different deductible periods. For example, the number of patients eligible for compensation in Colorado decreases from 5,919 to 1,604 with use of a four-week deductible period and to 973 with an eight-

Table 1.5. Cost Components of Swedish Compensable Events, with Eight-Week Deductible Period (in millions of dollars).

Type of Loss	Loss Total		1992 Value of Loss (%)	
	Utah	Colorado	Utah	Colorado
Income and household production				
Gross wage loss	21.35	31.49		
Fringe benefits	5.47	7.92		
Less:				
Taxes	−4.16	−6.90		
Consumption deduction	−2.36	−3.64		
Household production	−11.63	−7.14		
SSDI benefit	−1.65	−3.39		
Household production loss	44.02	52.03	45.78	57.51
Net income and household production loss	51.05	70.37	(59.6)	(57.5)

Health care costs						
Gross costs	21.58	49.99	19.63		45.12	
Less:						
Compensation from health insurance	−17.26	−40.00	−15.70		−36.10	
Net health care costs	4.32	9.99	3.93	(5.1)	9.02	(9.0)
Other compensable costs						
Burial expenses	2.08	1.25	2.08	(2.7)	1.25	(1.3)
Pain and suffering	25.00	32.21	25.00	(32.6)	32.21	(32.2)
Total compensable costs	**82.44**	**113.82**	**76.79**	**(100.0)**	**99.99**	**(100.0)**

Table 1.6. Affordability of Preferred No-Fault Models in Utah and Colorado (in millions, discounted to 1992 dollars).

State	Estimates of Preferred No-Fault Models	Current Malpractice System Costs
Utah	54.9[a]	55–60
Colorado	82.0[b]	100–110

[a] Based on use of Swedish compensable events; health care costs; $100,000 cap on pain and suffering; four-week disability period; no household production; 66% wage replacement. [b] Based on use of Swedish compensable events; health care costs; eight-week disability period; no household production; full wage replacement.

week period. Proportionally similar decreases occur in Utah when the same time thresholds are used.

More generally, Table 1.7 illustrates how the various components of the compensation package can be treated as modules. Policymakers could use precisely such methods to cost out alternative compensation schemes. Decisions about the trade-offs involved in design issues, such as numbers of patients eligible for compensation and the importance of household production to awards, could play out in public and legislative debates about appropriate uses of scarce resources. Of course these decisions go to the central problem of distributive justice in compensation. An administrative compensation scheme cannot circumvent the need to make difficult decisions about who and what types of injuries should receive compensation. However, it would (and does in the workers' compensation setting) allow stakeholders to agree on eligible injuries and obtainable remedies in advance, which we believe would promote equity, predictability, and efficiency in the distribution process.

Two other advantages of a no-fault approach warrant mention. First, if it were carefully designed, a no-fault scheme could eliminate much of the adversarial approach to medical malpractice litigation. We were astonished to find that physicians in Sweden actively participate in 60 to 80 percent of the claims that are made, helping their patients complete and file the relevant forms. Com-

Table 1.7. Economic Consequences of Swedish Compensable Events (in millions, discounted to 1992 dollars).

	Utah	Colorado
Any disability	(N = 2,940)	(N = 5,919)
Total	$90.90	$128.88
Less household production	60.38	90.55
Less household production and pain and suffering	27.16	38.51
>4 weeks disability	(N = 1,465)	(N = 1,604)
Total	$82.55	$84.23
Less household production	52.42	52.99
Less household production and pain and suffering	25.22	21.21
>8 weeks disability	(N = 889)	(N = 973)
Total	$76.78	$87.44
Less household production	45.96	52.18
Less household production and pain and suffering	20.96	19.97

pensation there appears to be culturally ingrained as a matter of social justice, not necessarily as an admission of provider guilt or negligence. Hence it tends to support rather than conflict with the health care professional's commitment to the patient and to excellence in medical practice. This milieu appears to be ascribable, at least in part, to the structural separation of insurance and disciplinary mechanisms.

Second, we believe that an avoidability-based compensation scheme could provide an enormous boost to error reduction efforts. As the Institute of Medicine's report has recently made clear, many errors fall into the avoidable category and could be reduced if proper error prevention strategies were put into place. There is also increasing recognition that the implementation and success of such strategies hinges on the free flow of information. The specter of litigation currently stands as a major barrier to the free flow of information about medical errors. Thus, removing it would align the foci of the compensation and quality improvement systems and center them on precisely those injuries that are eradicable.

Conclusion

The main objectives of the UCPMS were to test the results of the HMPS in another health care environment and to explore the feasibility of a no-fault system for compensating medical injury. With support from the Robert Wood Johnson Foundation; cooperation from hospitals, physicians, and malpractice insurers in Utah and Colorado; and the efforts of numerous collaborators, these objectives were achieved. Overall the UCMPS lent strong support to the iatrogenic injury rates, economic calculations, and malpractice patterns estimated in New York nearly a decade earlier. The UCMPS findings were no carbon copy, however. For instance, we found significantly lower iatrogenic death rates in Utah and Colorado. We also gained fresh insights into the burden of iatrogenic injury by investigating several previously understudied areas, such as the resources devoted to outpatient services to treat the morbidity caused by adverse events.

The results of our efforts to conceptualize and cost out an administrative compensation scheme based on avoidability criteria provide considerable cause for optimism about the feasibility of a no-fault system. Even before our work was complete, however, it was apparent in both states that the enthusiasm of our collaborators would not be sufficient to transform the no-fault initiative into political action. The 1990s malpractice crisis that many pundits envisioned, owing to the experience of the two previous decades, did not eventuate, and relative stability in malpractice insurance markets appeared to sap legislative interest in large-scale tort reform.

Thus skeptics would have some foundation for concluding that the true mission of the UCMPS failed; a key part of its empirical findings has not generated policy reform. We prefer to take a longer-term view of the value of the study. It is our hope that when the political winds shift, a probable occurrence given a history of cyclical interest in alternative compensation approaches in the United States, the UCMPS methods and findings will stand ready to be used by those policymakers who become newly interested in a no-fault approach.

Hints of just such a shift have surfaced at the federal level over the past six months. Ironically, rather than being born of dissatisfaction with the malpractice system as a mechanism for compensating injured patients, interest in malpractice alternatives has been invigorated by a spate of media and political attention directed at error in medicine. As optimal strategies for reducing medical error continue to emphasize the need for open communication about mistakes and attention to systemic, not individual, fault, new light is being cast on the merits of a different approach to medical injury compensation.

Notes

1. Note, however, that this phenomenon does not necessarily lend support to views about greedy personal injury lawyers and vexatious plaintiffs. "[I]t is more likely due to the fact," Weiler (1995) argues, "that (previously ill) patients and their lawyers have a difficult time identifying in advance valid claims that demonstrate that something went wrong in treatment" (p. 1162).

2. These percentages relate to the proportion of drug-related events due to negligence, not drug-related adverse events in general.

3. QAHCS investigators did not make determinations about negligence. Instead, physician reviewers were asked to determine whether each adverse event detected was "preventable," defined as "an error in management due to failure to follow accepted practice at an individual or system level" (Wilson et al., 1995, p. 458).

4. Chief among these differences is the fact that Andrews and colleagues focused on surgery—precisely the area where we had detected the highest rates of adverse events in the general hospital population we examined.

5. A deductible, or threshold, period of this kind is a device for eliminating relatively nonserious injuries from the pool of injuries eligible
for compensation. It also has the benefit of channeling available funds
to victims whose losses are least likely to be covered by other sources
of coverage, such as sick pay for time lost from work (see Haas, 1987).

References

Abraham, K., & Weiler, P. C. (1994). Enterprise liability and the evolution of
the American health care system. *Harvard Law Review, 108*, 381–486.

Abramson, E. M. (1989–1990). The medical malpractice imbroglio: A non-
adversarial suggestion. *Kentucky Law Journal, 78*, 293–310.

Anderson, R. E. (1996). An "epidemic" of medical malpractice? A commentary
on the Harvard Medical Practice Study. *Civil Justice Memorandum*
(Vol. 27). New York: Manhattan Institute Center.

Andrews, L. B., Stocking, C., Krizek, T., Gottlieb, L., Krizek, C., Vargish, T.,
& Siegler, M. (1997, February 1). An alternative strategy for studying
adverse events in medical care. *Lancet 349*, 309–313.

Bates, D. W., Spell, N., Cullen, D. J., Burdick, E., Laird, N., Petersen, L. A.,
Small, S. D., Sweitzer, B. J., & Leape, L. L. (1997). The costs of adverse
drug events in hospitalized patients. *Journal of the American Medical Association, 277*, 307–311.

Bovbjerg, R. R. (1993). Medical malpractice: Research and reform. *Virginia Law
Review, 79*, 2155–2208.

Brennan, T. A. (1998). The role of regulation in quality improvement. *Milbank
Quarterly, 76*, 709, 714–716.

Brennan, T. A., Leape, L. L., Laird, N. M., Herbert, L. E., Localio, A. R.,
Lawthers, A. G., Newhouse, J. P., Weiler, P. C., & Hiatt, H. H. (1991).
Incidence of adverse events and negligence in hospitalized patients:
Results of the Harvard Medical Practice Study I. *New England Journal
of Medicine, 324*, 370–376.

Brennan, T. A., Localio, A. R., & Laird, N. M. (1989). Reliability and validity
of judgments concerning adverse events suffered by hospitalized patients.
Medical Care, 27, 1148–1158.

Burstin, H. R., Johnson, W. G., Lipsitz, S. R., & Brennan, T. A. (1993). Do the
poor sue more? *Journal of the American Medical Association, 270*, 1697–
1710.

California Medical Association & California Hospital Association. (1977).
Report on the Medical Insurance Feasibility Study (Don H. Mills, Ed.). San
Francisco, Sutter.

Classen, D. C., Pestotnik, S. L., Evans, R. S., Lloyd, J. F., & Burke, J. P. (1997). Adverse drug events in hospitalized patients: Excess length-of-stay, extra costs, and attributable mortality. *Journal of the American Medical Association, 277,* 301–306.

Danzon, P. M. (1985). *Medical malpractice: Theory, evidence, and public policy.* Cambridge, MA: Harvard University Press.

Gandhi, T. K., Burstin, H. R., Cook, E. F., Puopolo, A. L., Haas, J. S., Brennan, T. A., & Bates, D. W. (2000). Drug complications in outpatients. *Journal of General Internal Medicine, 15,* 149–154.

Gawande, A. A., Thomas, E. J., Zinner, M. J., & Brennan, T. A. (1999). The incidence and nature of surgical adverse events in Colorado and Utah in 1992. *Surgery, 126,* 66–75.

Haas, T. F. (1987). On reintegrating workers' compensation and employers' liability. *Georgia Law Review, 21,* 843–898.

Harvard Medical Practice Study. (1990). *Patients, doctors, and lawyers: Medical injury, malpractice litigation, and patient compensation in New York.* Cambridge, MA: President and Fellows of Harvard College.

Havighurst, C. C., & Tancredi, L. R. (1973). Medical adversity insurance: A no-fault approach to medical malpractice and quality assurance. *Milbank Quarterly, 51,* 125–168.

Hayward, R. A., Bernard, A. M., Rosevear, J. S., Anderson, J. E., & McMahon, L. F. (1993). An evaluation of generic screens for poor quality of hospital care on a general medicine service. *Medical Care, 31,* 394–402.

Hofer, T. P., Berstein, S. J., De Monner, S., & Hayward, R. A. (2000). Discussion between reviewers does not improve reliability of peer review of hospital quality. *Medical Care, 38,* 152–161.

Johnson, W. G., Brennan, T. A., Newhouse, J. P., Leape, L. L., Lawthers, A. G., Hiatt, H. H., & Weiler, P. C. (1992). The economic consequences of medical injuries. *Journal of the American Medical Association, 267,* 2478–2492.

Kohn, L. T., Corrigan, J. M., & Donaldson, M. S. (Eds.); Committee on Quality of Health Care in America, Institute of Medicine. (2000). *To err is human: Building a safer health system.* Washington, DC: National Academy Press.

Leape, L. L. (1994). Error in medicine. *Journal of the American Medical Association, 272,* 1851–1857.

Leape, L. L. (1998). Promoting patient safety by preventing medical error. *Journal of the American Medical Association, 280,* 1444–1447.

Legal Services Corporation Act. (1999). 45 C.F.R. § 1609 ("Fee-Generating Cases").

Levit, K. R., Lazenby, H. C., Cowan, C. A., Won, D. K., Stiller, J. M., Sivarajan, L., & Stewart, M. W. (1995). State health expenditure accounts: Building blocks for state health spending analysis. *Health Care Financing Review*, *17*, 201–254.

Liang, B. A. (1999). Error in medicine: Legal impediments to U.S. reform. *Journal of Health Politics Policy & Law*, *24*, 27–58.

Localio, A. R., Lawthers, A. G., Brennan, T. A., Laird, N. M., Herbert, L. E., Peterson, L. M., Newhouse, J. P., Weiler, P. C., & Hiatt, H. H. (1991). Relation between malpractice claims and adverse events to negligence: Results of the Harvard Medical Practice Study III. *New England Journal of Medicine*, *325*, 245–251.

Localio, A. R., Weaver, S. L., Landis, J. R., Lawthers, A. G., Brennan, T. A., Herbert, L. E., & Sharp, T. J. (1996). Identifying adverse events caused by medical care: Degree of physician agreement in a retrospective chart review. *Annals of Internal Medicine*, *125*, 457–464.

Mashaw, J. L., & Marmor, T. R. (1994). Conceptualizing, estimating, and reforming fraud, waste, and abuse in health care spending. *Yale Journal on Regulation*, *11*, 455–494.

McNulty, M. (1989). Are poor patients likely to sue for malpractice? *Journal of the American Medical Association*, *262*, 1391–1392.

Mills, D. H. (1978, April). Medical Insurance Feasibility Study: A technical summary. *Western Journal of Medicine*, *128*, 360–365.

O'Connell, J. (1975). No-fault insurance for injuries arising from medical treatment: A proposal for elective coverage. *Emory Law Journal*, *24*, 21.

Oldertz, C. (1998). The patient, pharmaceutical and security insurances. In C. Oldertz & E. Tidefelt (Eds.), *Compensation for personal injury in Sweden and 17 other countries*. Philadelphia: Coronet Books.

Prosser, W., Keeton, W. P., and Dobbs, D. B. (1984). *Prosser & Keeton on the law of torts* (5th ed.). St. Paul, MN: West.

Rosenthal, M. M. (1987). *Dealing with medical malpractice: The British and Swedish experience*. London: Tavistock.

Sage, W. M., Hastings, K. E., & Berenson R. A. (1994). Enterprise liability for medical malpractice and health care quality improvement. *American Journal of Law & Medicine*, *20*, 1–36.

Saks, M. J. (1992). Do we really know anything about the behavior of the tort litigation system: And why not? *University of Pennsylvania Law Review*, *140*, 1147–1292.

Saks, M. J. (1994). Medical malpractice: Facing real problems and finding real solutions. *William & Mary Law Review*, *35*, 693–726.

Studdert, D. M., Thomas, E. J., Burstin, H. R., Zbar, B.I.W., Orav, J., & Brennan, T. A. (2000). Negligent care and malpractice claiming behavior in Utah and Colorado. *Medical Care, 38,* 250–260.

Studdert, D. M., Thomas, E. J., Zbar, B.I.W., Newhouse, J. P., Weiler, P. C., Bayuk, J., & Brennan, T. A. (1997, Spring). Can the United States afford a "no-fault" system of compensation for medical injury? *Law and Contemporary Problems, 60,* 1–34.

Sugarman, S. D. (1985). Doing away with tort law. *California Law Review, 73,* 558–664.

Sugarman, S. D. (1991). Doctor No. *University of Chicago Law Review, 58,* 1499–1516.

Taragin, M. I., Willet, L. R., Wilczek, A. P., Trout, R., & Carson, J. L. (1992). The influence of standard of care and severity of injury on the resolution of medical malpractice claims. *Annals of Internal Medicine, 117,* 780–784.

Thomas, E. J., Studdert, D. M., Newhouse, J. P., Zbar, B.I.W., Howard, K. M., Williams, E. J., & Brennan, T. A. (1999). Costs of medical injuries in Colorado and Utah in 1992. *Inquiry, 36,* 255–264.

Thomas, E. J., Studdert, D. M., Burstin, H. R., Orav, J., Zeena, T., Williams, E. J., Howard, K. M., Weiler, P. C., & Brenner, T. A. (2000a). Incidence and types of adverse events and negligent care in Utah and Colorado. *Medical Care, 38,* 261–271.

Thomas, E. J., Studdert, D. M., Runciman, W. B., Webb, R. K., Septon, E. J., Wilson, R. M., Gibberd, R. W., Harrison, B. T., & Brennan, T. A. (2000b). A comparison of iatrogenic injury studies in Australia and America II: Context, methods, casemix, population, patient and hospital characteristics. *International Journal for Quality in Health Care, 12,* 371–378.

Weiler, P. C. (1993). The case for no-fault medical liability. *Maryland Law Review, 52,* 908–949.

Weiler, P. C. (1995). Fixing the tail: The place of malpractice in health care reform. *Rutgers Law Review, 47,* 1157–1193.

Weiler, P. C., Hiatt, H. H., Newhouse, J. P., Johnson, W. G., Brennan, T. A., & Leape, L. L. (1993). *A measure of malpractice: Medical injury, malpractice litigation, and patient compensation.* Cambridge, MA: Harvard University Press.

White, M. J. (1994, Fall). The value of liability in medical malpractice. *Health Affairs,* pp. 75–87.

Wilson, R. M., Runciman, W. B., Gibberd, R. W., Harrison, B. T., Newby, L., and Hamilton, J. D. (1995, November 6). The Quality in Australian Health Care Study. *Medical Journal of Australia, 163,* 458–471.

Part Two

Error from the Perspective
of Providers and Patients

One of the most striking aspects in the study of medical mishaps is the importance of perspective and definition.

Physicians and patients perceive an incident from different perspectives and describe it with different language. Furthermore, different specialties face quite different mishap situations. Nurses, for example, are vulnerable to their own errors in their roles as important clinicians but they are also witnesses to physician error.

Part Two (Chapters Two through Five) provides a glimpse into the perspective of a transplant surgeon who suspects that stress and burnout are key factors in surgical errors but frets that the evidence is anecdotal rather than empirical. An academic primary care doctor considers the extent to which the hospital-oriented discussions in *To Err Is Human* can be applied to ambulatory care settings. A chief of nursing describes the implicit "code of silence" about errors that physicians and nurses share. She suggests that this tacit code adds to the difficulty of understanding the nature and incidence of error. Finally, a journalist describes the patient's perspective, highlighting the media's role (both useful and destructive) in bringing cases of mishaps to the public's attention, and reminding us of the patient's frustration when trying to get information.

Part Two hints at the confusion that arises from differing choices of words and differing definitions that bedevil the study of error.

When discussing undesirable outcomes, physicians prefer terms like *adverse event*, *known risk*, *unexpected complications*, words that reflect the uncertainties in medical practice and its probabilistic nature. The profession of medicine defines *error* and *mistake* more narrowly than does the public.

Suffice it to say that reaching agreement about what we are studying and preventing will be a high priority in the next wave of research and national discussion.

2

How Stress and Burnout Produce Medical Mistakes

Darrell A. Campbell Jr. and Patricia L. Cornett

Increasing scrutiny by the public, the health care profession, and the government is leading to more intense examination into the causes and conditions that produce medical mistakes. The 1999 Institute of Medicine study *To Err Is Human* focused public attention on this issue and its grave consequences for patients, physicians, nurses, health care administrators, and all those involved in providing or receiving medical care in hospitals today (Kohn, Corrigan, & Donaldson, 2000). The intent of the Institute of Medicine study was not to lay blame on individuals or institutions but to offer recommendations for reforming the system. Its goals were to change the circumstances in which medical errors are likely to occur and, by so doing, to improve patient safety and reduce the risk of deadly medical mistakes.

Health care practitioners have been aware of the gravity of this problem for at least a decade (Leape, 1996; Firth-Cozens, 1993). For example, two 1991 Harvard Medical Practice Studies evaluated the incidence and nature of *adverse events*—what we are calling *medical mistakes*—in more than 30,000 randomly selected New York State medical records. The first study (Brennan et al., 1991) reviewed the association between these adverse events (defined as injuries caused by medical management) and negligence or substandard care. Of the 3.7 percent of adverse events that resulted in hospitalizations, 27.6 percent were due to negligence, a rate that was significantly higher among the elderly. The second study (Leape et al., 1991) examined these adverse events in terms of type of error, association with negligence, and degree of disability. More than half (58 percent) were due to errors in management, and nearly half of those were attributed to negligence. Adverse events during surgery were less likely to be caused by negligence (17 percent) than were non-surgical ones (37 percent). The proportion of adverse events due to negligence was highest for diagnostic mishaps (75 percent); non-invasive therapeutic mishaps, or *errors of omission* (77 percent); and events occurring in the emergency room (70 percent) (Leape et al., 1991; Leape, 1996).

The authors of these Harvard Medical Practice Studies concluded that many such medical mistakes are preventable. They urged that reducing the incidence of such negligence means identifying the systematic causes and consequences of medical mistakes and developing methods to reduce their frequency and severity. Their findings "represent an agenda for research on quality of care" (Leape et al., 1991, p. 383).

This chapter responds to that agenda by examining the psychological and workplace factors that create an environment in which physicians, in particular surgeons, are more likely to make serious medical mistakes. Our contention is that the high levels of stress and burnout experienced by surgeons not only negatively affect their clinical performance and social interactions but also create an environment conducive to medical mistakes. The connection may be subtle and indirect, but it is nevertheless real.

When the connection between environmental stress and medical mistakes has been explored at all, it has been from the perspective of medical malpractice. The 1988 study of Jones et al. on stress and medical malpractice found a moderate to strong association between a stressful workplace and the risk of malpractice and carried that connection to its inevitable litigious conclusion: "workplace and personal stress adversely affect physical, cognitive, and affective functioning, thus impairing health care judgments, decision making, and behaviors that lead to malpractice" (p. 728).

Considerable literature in the last twenty years has examined the relationship between stress and burnout on job performance. Stressors, or conditions that negatively impact job performance, have been identified (Cohen, 1980; Campbell, 1999). These conditions exactly mirror those that surgeons experience routinely every day. It is no surprise that many studies with different experimental designs all support the view that physicians and other health care workers have higher levels of stress and burnout than other professionals (Campbell, 1999; Felton, 1998; Kahill, 1988; Leiter, 1991; Weinberg & Creed, 2000).

For example, Kahill (1988) reviewed the ten-year evidence (from 1974 to 1984) of burnout among nurses, mental health workers, and other health care professionals. Firth-Cozens (1993, p. 136) concurred that levels of stress, depression, and addiction are higher among doctors than in the general population. More recently, Weinberg and Creed (2000, p. 533) reported that between 25 percent and 50 percent of the U.K. National Health Service staff reported job-related stress. These authors used a case control design to determine the link between stress on and off the job and anxiety and depressive disorders among physicians, nurses, and administrative and ancillary health care workers.

The dry statistics of these reports can be dramatized more vividly by considering the hypothetical example of Dr. I. M. Weary, a third-year surgical resident. Although this example is fictitious, it is representative of countless real-life scenarios and is supported by a wealth of statistics and data about the demands on today's surgical resident (as cited, for example, in Campbell, 1999; also see Samkoff & Jacques, 1991; Orton & Gruzelier, 1989; Deary & Tait, 1987).

A Day in the Life of a Stressed Surgical Resident, or, How Dr. I. M. Weary Made a Medical Mistake

Dr. Weary has just been summoned to the emergency room to place a chest tube in a trauma patient. It is 10 P.M. and the ER is crowded and noisy. Swarms of white coats buzz from one bed to the next, phones ring, alarms blare, and nurses bark out orders. While he is evaluating his patient, Dr. Weary's beeper goes off at three inopportune intervals. One of his calls is trivial but annoying; one involves a patient with a serious problem in the surgical intensive care unit; and one, possibly the most alarming, reminds Dr. Weary that he is scheduled to present a case to 150 surgeons at the death and complications conference on the following morning (Dr. Weary does not enjoy public speaking).

His task is at hand, however, and Dr. Weary must concentrate his attention on placing a rather large chest tube—safely, calmly, and gently—between the patient's ribs into the thoracic cavity.

But Dr. Weary makes a serious mistake: he places the chest tube below the level of the diaphragm and thus into the abdominal cavity, rather than into the thoracic cavity as he had intended. When the error is discovered, he lashes out at the patient (for moving), at the nurse (for not providing proper lighting and equipment), and at the patient's family as well. On the surface this complication is related to Dr. Weary's level of skill, training, and knowledge. These qualities would certainly be scrutinized in a court of law if litigation ensued. But what about some of the other, less tangible factors that come into play in this scenario?

Burnout

One of the factors that could seriously affect Dr. Weary's interest in and motivation for performing quality service is a condition referred to as *burnout*. Several definitions of burnout can be found in the psychological literature; the three-part definition of Maslach is one that is widely accepted (Kahill, 1988, p. 284; Leiter, 1991, p. 549). The three components are emotional exhaustion, depersonalization, and reduced personal accomplishment (Maslach & Jackson, 1986; Kahill, 1988, p. 284; Campbell, 1999, p. 602). Maslach's instrument for measuring burnout, the Maslach Burnout Inventory, defines it as "a state of emotional exhaustion in which service providers view recipients impersonally and their own performance disparagingly" (Leiter, 1991, p. 549).

Maslach's definition precisely mirrors the daily situation of the practicing clinician in today's medical environment. The workload demands that stress the physician are well known and amply documented. Felton (1998), for example, systematically reviewed the weight of studies showing how the greater demands placed on the modern physician result in higher levels of stress and burnout. At the same time, the traditional high respect accorded the medical profession has been seriously eroded, further contributing to stress and burnout.

Limited resources are another stressor. As hospitals and departments close, as staffs and budgets are slashed, those who remain on the job experience greater demands for their services and suffer high levels of stress. A series of articles in the *Detroit News* (see, for example, Webster, 2000) described the frustration experienced by doctors as well as their patients when three Detroit area hospitals closed because of Medicare and Medicaid cuts. One article vividly reported the struggles of the staff at St. John Riverview Hospital in metropolitan Detroit to cope with heavier caseloads and reduced resources. Since the closure of other nearby hospitals, visits to the emergency room at Riverview have increased 30 to 40 percent, and urgent lab tests that should be done immediately now take six hours.

Frustration over having to deal with these stressors increases the risk of burnout. Exhaustion with the failure of the usual coping mechanisms, both personal and professional, leads to discouragement and disenchantment, attitudes that ultimately lead to cynicism and even despair. These negative moods inevitably result in reduced accomplishment (Maslach's third component) and loss of job effectiveness. The costs are turnover, absenteeism, and physical illness, including substance abuse. Other costs are the deterioration in the physician's relationship with patients and coworkers. Perhaps the most dramatic cost is the high rate of suicide among individuals in the health care field—twice as high as in other professions (Felton, 1998, p. 241; Pilowski & O'Sullivan, 1989, p. 269). It is not hard to imagine that feelings of emotional exhaustion and disenchantment could lead to a lack of focus, with disastrous results for the patient.

Relationship Between Stress, Burnout, and Job Performance

Several decades of work in experimental psychology (Cohen, 1980; Leiter, 1991; Firth-Cozens, 1993; Felton, 1998; Kahill, 1988) have documented how these stressors can affect job performance in more subtle ways. Investigations into the relationship between stressor and performance have determined that stress may have an effect on performance even though the stressor itself has terminated. Selye described this phenomenon as an *adaptive cost* relationship, in which prolonged exposure to a stressor requires progressive adaptation to the stress and leads ultimately to exhaustion (Cohen, 1980, pp. 82–83). Many subsequent studies have examined the types of stress that reliably produce poststress performance effects. These data indicate that the aftereffects of stress may influence performance and that predictability, control, crowding, and task load are important variables affecting this relationship. Although there is a danger in stretching the point too far, many of the stressful aspects of Dr. Weary's experience bear a parallel to experimental variables studied in this context.

Predictability

Some of the most interesting stressor variables involve *predictability*, a variable in short supply in the medical environment. Uncertainty about outcomes is at the core of modern medical practice. Dittus, Roberts, and Wilson (1989) have described some of the factors surrounding uncertainty in medical decision making: ambiguity of relevant data, lack of understanding of basic biological processes, and the need to act before all information can be gathered. As a result, "uncertainty produces great anxiety for both the decision maker and the patient because it generally means that there is a chance of a bad outcome as well as a good one" and "even the best decision can result in a bad outcome" (p. 23A). Anderson, Jay, Weng, and Anderson (1995, p. 869) have described clinical uncertainty as technical, personal, or conceptual. *Technical* uncertainty results from the lack of scientific data to predict clinical outcomes. *Personal* uncertainty refers to the physician's ignorance of the patient's values, attitudes, and concerns. *Conceptual* uncertainty occurs when the physician applies abstract knowledge to practical clinical situations. As a result of their study of physicians using a diagnostic expert system, these investigators concluded that the stress of dealing with clinical uncertainty has a negative effect on physicians' clinical performance.

In a typical psychological experiment to test the effect of unpredictability on stress levels, subjects were exposed to unpredictable bursts of noise (conglomerate noise made up of typical urban sounds). Immediately after the noise was stopped, the subjects were asked to perform a standard *tolerance for frustration* task involving sequential exposure to four puzzles, two of which could be solved and two of which could not. When compared with controls (subjects exposed to continuous uninterrupted noise), those exposed to the unpredictable noise stressor tended to give up earlier on the insoluble puzzles; that is, they showed a lower tolerance for frustration in the poststress performance measure (Cohen, 1980, pp. 83–84).

Control

Control is always an issue in medical practice, especially for those in positions of lesser authority or autonomy (nurses, for example). But all health care workers in today's world of managed care and insurance restrictions experience the loss of control and autonomy (Leiter, 1991). In experiments, lack of control of the stressor is an important variable that can produce important poststress effects. Classic experiments demonstrated that subjects exposed to noise performed better than other subjects on postnoise tolerance to frustration testing when they were told that they could terminate the noise exposure by pushing a button, even if they did not actually do so. The other subjects exposed to the noise had no such control (Cohen, 1980, p. 91). By extrapolation, Dr. Weary might have had a better chance of placing the chest tube correctly if he had perceived that he could quit and go home after he first walked into the ER, even though he probably would have been fired if he had done so.

Conversely, research has clearly shown that greater control and autonomy are consistently associated with lower levels of burnout (Leiter, 1991, p. 553). Interestingly, even indirect control seems to have an ameliorating effect on poststressor performance (Cohen, 1980, p. 93). Subjects exposed to noise performed better on poststress measures when they had information that a partner could terminate the noise exposure even though they themselves could not. Likewise, control over initiating the noise stressor was a variable that resulted in improved poststress performance. Before performance testing, subjects were told that they could elect to avoid noise exposure although the examiner would prefer that they be exposed to the noise. The subjects invariably acquiesced, but their postnoise performance testing results were better than those of controls who were not given the same option (Cohen, 1980, p. 91).

Crowding

The social density of the environment is also a stressor that seems to affect performance. At 10 P.M. the ER of most large hospitals would be an ideal venue to study this situation, although solving puzzles and placing chest tubes are two very different performance measures. The experimental data, nevertheless, indicate that *crowding* affects performance. For example, eight high school girls were asked to perform simple tasks for one hour in a small or a large room. Afterward the tolerance for frustration test was administered. Subjects who worked in the crowded environment (small room) had less tolerance for frustration than did subjects who had worked in the uncrowded environment (Cohen, 1980, pp. 87, 94).

Task Load

The strain on the resources of staff, time, and dollars in modern hospitals also affects the *task load* of health care providers. Fewer are required to do more with less (Meyerson, 1990, p. 974). Some aspects of task load also seem to affect performance. In experiments where the stressor involved reaction to one hundred lights, subjects showed reduced tolerance for frustration on poststress performance testing when compared with subjects who had been asked to respond to only fifty lights. In another instance, in what might seem to most of us to be a particularly evil experimental design, subjects who were asked to perform a task were also told they might be called upon to recall a speech, even though this follow-up never actually happened. But in those subjects who had to worry about the possibility of giving a speech, tolerance for frustration was reduced poststress (Cohen, 1980, p. 89). Thinking about next morning's D&C conference, Dr. Weary might well have considered this onerous prospect as he prepared to examine his patient.

Psychological Basis for the Relationship Between Stress and Job Performance

The psychological basis for the relationship between stress and subsequent job performance has been a subject of great interest. Three theories lend themselves particularly well to a consideration of how stress could predispose health care professionals to medical mistakes. The *cognitive fatigue* hypothesis posits that prolonged stress results in the contraction of *attentional capacity*, because all such attentional resources have been devoted to the stressor itself, with little capacity left for the performance. This theory is supported by studies demonstrating that poststress performance suffers when the task load is higher.

Back in the ER, therefore, Dr. Weary's attentional reserves might well have been depleted by incessant pages and other patient care concerns — not to mention his imminent presentation at the D&C conference! As a result, an important detail is missed, and a serious error is made in placing the chest tube in the patient. A more global way to think about cognitive fatigue is to view it as what occurs when a physician functions in an environment of information overload, which is an undeniable aspect of modern medical practice.

Learned helplessness is another theory that could apply to the performance problems encountered in the medical environment. According to this theory the subject learns over time that a response does not influence the stressor, and ultimately he or she loses the motivation needed to perform a subsequent task. Finally, the *frustration mood* hypothesis holds that progressive frustration with the stressor leads to sufficient annoyance and irritation that performance on subsequent tasks is diminished and interpersonal relations are adversely affected as well.

The underlying mechanism, whether it be cognitive fatigue, learned helplessness, or frustration mood effect, undoubtedly depends to some extent on the individual involved, but each theory may help to explain how a well-trained and well-meaning professional could be influenced by a stressful environment in such a way that performance is affected and a medical mishap occurs.

Relationship Between Stress, Burnout, and Social Interactions

Besides its negative effect on job performance, stress also takes a heavy toll on social interactions. In a classic experimental study illustrating the effects of stress on depersonalization, subjects were taken to a supermarket and asked to find various items, the variables being density of the shopping area and task load. Following the shopping task, subjects were asked to meet the examiner, but instead they encountered an individual who had apparently lost a contact lens. Subjects who had been exposed to a high task load or crowded conditions were less apt to help the unfortunate individual than were the appropriate controls (Cohen & Spacapan, 1978). Similar experiments using a noise as a stressor demonstrated increased aggression and competitiveness following various stressors.

These observations are highly relevant to a discussion about stress in the medical environment because caring for the sick, diseased, and distressed is a central feature of the professional code of conduct for health care workers. These experiments also bear on the major performance measure of any medical institution, the effective doctor-patient relationship. Consequently, depersonalization, one of the three components of the Maslach Burnout Inventory, is more critical in the health care field than in most other professions (Leiter, 1991). In all instances, it negatively affects the relationship of the caregiver with patients and coworkers. Depersonalization can take many forms, ranging from passive withdrawal from social and professional relationships to callous disregard for the needs of clients to active violence against those for whom the health worker is responsible. All of these reactions have been documented in many studies (Deckard, Meterko, & Field, 1994, p. 752; Kahill, 1988, p. 289).

Other Conditions and Factors That Contribute to Stress and Burnout

In addition to being particularly subject to these proven stressors, medical professionals often work under extreme conditions of fatigue and sleep deprivation, information complexity and mental overload, and organizational stress.

Fatigue and Sleep Deprivation

Research over the last several decades has documented the detrimental effects on job performance of fatigue and loss of sleep among workers who are "hazarding the night" (1994). For example, Krueger (1989) summarized the research findings on reductions in sustained performance resulting from fatigue, especially during and following one or more nights of complete sleep loss or longer periods of reduced or fragmented sleep. He concluded: "sleep loss appears to result in reduced reaction time, decreased vigilance, perceptual and cognitive distortions, and changes in affect. Sleep loss and workload interact with circadian rhythms in producing their effects" (p. 129). Although the early studies, like those reviewed by Krueger, were performed in the technical and aerospace industries, these findings were soon extended to the health care field, specifically to medical residents and house officers (Samkoff & Jacques, 1991; Orton & Gruzelier, 1989; Deary & Tait, 1987; Firth-Cozens, 1993).

The 1991 review by Samkoff and Jacques brought out several results that are relevant to our thesis in this chapter. Among the trends they noted was an increase in negative moods. Hostility and anger were greater in residents after one night's sleep loss and in those in the midyear of their training compared with those at the start of training. The implications of this trend for the quality of the doctor-patient relationship have been discussed in several reports, but no study has yet examined it systematically. Symptoms of depression were also commonly reported after acute and chronic sleep deprivation. Firth-Cozens (1993, p. 138) reported similar findings. In her study of junior medical house officers, the number of hours of sleep during the previous forty-eight hours and levels of stress were significantly correlated, as were sleep patterns and both stress and depression.

The findings from both these reviews about the effects of fatigue and sleep deprivation on measures of performance were less conclusive. Firth-Cozens (p. 140) noted that the negative effect of sleep deprivation on performance seems to vary with the intrinsic interest of the task and with individual factors. However, Samkoff and Jacques (1991) noted that clinical tasks requiring sustained vigilance or concentration were the most sensitive to deterioration after sleep loss and fatigue. Given their findings, they agreed with the recommendations of the Association of American Medical Colleges to limit the total working hours for residents to no more than eighty hours per week averaged over four weeks.

Information Complexity and Mental Overload

The technological world of the late twentieth century has given all of us many benefits unknown to our ancestors one or two generations ago. Even ten years ago, who had even heard of the Internet or the World Wide Web? Or who could have imagined what impact these electronic technologies would have on our personal and professional lives? But one cost of these advances has been an increasing complexity in both the quantity and quality of available information and options. We have already discussed briefly the negative effect of uncertainty and ambiguity on medical decision making. One new contributor to uncertainty is the sheer complexity of information the modern physician can access with a keystroke and must bring to bear on the decision-making process. It might seem that having more and better information would enhance the physician's ability to make an informed decision about the best care for a patient. Indeed, that is often the case. Just as often, however, too much information, especially complex information, produces mental overload and creates stress on the human capacity to process information effectively.

A relevant illustration of this paradox was reported in a recent study of medical decision making by Redelmeier and Shafir (1995). When family physicians were presented with multiple medication options for a patient with osteoarthritis, they were less likely to prescribe a drug when they had to decide between two different medications than they were when they were given only one drug choice. Evidently, the difficulty of having to decide between two drugs had the paradoxical effect of keeping the physicians from choosing any medication at all.

Psychologists have studied such limitations on information processing for many years, and their findings have been applied to personnel in the military and technical fields (Svensson, Angelborg-Thanderz, Sjöberg, & Olsson, 1997; Stern & Keller, 1991). According to this research, when the individual is presented with too many alternatives with too many attributes, all competing for attention simultaneously, mental overload results. Humans cannot distinguish between more than six or seven discrete entities at the same time or hold more than that number in their short-term memory. Seven elements appear to be the maximum number for reliable decision making in uncertain situations (Svensson et al., 1997, pp. 362–363).

When Svensson et al. (1997) applied these psychological findings to a study of pilot performance and decision making, they found that even moderately complex information interfered with the pilots' ability to perform flight tasks (p. 377). The mental workload was affected by the complexity of the information, which also affected other aspects of performance. Interestingly, pilots who were more alert, active, relaxed, and confident before the tests were better able to cope with the mental load (p. 378). The authors noted that in relation to performance, mood dimensions such as hedonic tone, activation, tension, and control have predictive power. Their results accord with the scientific literature on human information processing. Conclusions about the relationship between the limitations of human information processing and the expansive possibilities of technological advancements are worth noting. As Svensson et al. (1997) noted, "the limit of performance is set by the limitations of the human operator and not by technological possibilities" (p. 378). Aircraft designers, in other words, need to join with specialists in human factors analysis (discussed later in this chapter) to design systems that work synchronously with the limits of the human ability to process information.

Organizational Stress

Organizational stress may be manifested in two distinct but related ways. On one hand, individuals in the medical environment may experience stress because of negative features of the organizational structure in which they work. On the other hand, as Firth-Cozens (1993, p. 143) succinctly puts it, "whole organizations can also be described as stressed, sick, or neurotic." Although a symbiotic relationship no doubt exists between these two manifestations, it may be going too far to say that an organization with many stressed workers is also likely to be a "sick" organization.

Most recent research in this area has focused on the first aspect of organizational stress on individual health care workers. Perhaps the most obvious example derives from the bureaucratic structure of managed care and the increased demands and restraints it places on the physician. In one such study surveying physicians in two staff-model health maintenance organizations (HMOs), Deckard et al. (1994) assessed the relationship between physician burnout and personal, professional, and organizational/worklife factors. Over half of the physicians (58 percent) reported high emotional exhaustion, and the highest predictors were the factors of workload/ scheduling and input/influence. The former included the amount of time physicians were on call, the amount of time allotted for administrative and committee work and paperwork, and the daily load of patients to be seen. The latter factor involved the amount of input, autonomy, or control the physician had over the policies and practices of the HMO (p. 751).

Leiter's work (1991) in this area emphasizes the importance of autonomy and control in ameliorating high levels of burnout among human service professionals. In mental health and medical settings, workers who could participate in organizational decisions had consistently lower levels of burnout than those who had no such opportunity (p. 553). For Leiter, "burnout is a sign of problems in the organizational context of human service professions" (p. 554).

Relationship Between Burnout and Stress and Medical Mistakes

The conclusion seems inescapable that there is a strong association between high levels of stress and burnout among health care workers and their organizations and an increased propensity to commit medical mistakes of all kinds. However, the evidence marshaled throughout this chapter to support this conclusion is largely circumstantial and indirect. Testing this conclusion in controlled studies has yet to be done on a large scale. Perhaps the next stage of research in this field will be devoted to just such studies.

One model that has been developed to test this conclusion is the insurance malpractice claim model. Jones (1988) reported the results of several studies by industrial psychologists in which there was a statistically significant correlation between hospitals whose employees reported high levels of stress on a human factors inventory and a higher frequency and severity of malpractice claims. Employees of these hospitals had the following characteristics: they all perceived a lack of support from management; they engaged in counterproductive, harmful on-the-job activities (for example, alcohol or drug abuse); and they reported high levels of job dissatisfaction and emotional distress. This study also included intervention in the form of a one-year hospitalwide stress management program. After one year, the number of malpractice claims dropped by 76 percent and 54 percent over the two previous years (p. 76).

Another approach to ameliorating stress is *human factors analysis*. This field developed after World War II in the military, aerospace, and nuclear industries (Fleger, 1993; LaBar, 1996; Stern & Keller, 1991). It focuses on the role of humans and human error in the workplace, but takes a systems approach in which the worker is one of several key elements in the system. The goal of human factors analysis is to design new systems or redesign existing systems in order to minimize human error, reduce the number of accidents, and improve efficiency. *Human factors* and *ergonomics* are terms often used interchangeably, but the former tends to focus on the mental aspects of performing a task whereas the latter is concerned primarily with the physical demands of a job (LaBar, 1996, p. 49).

Although human factors analysis has proved to be an effective approach in these technical industries, the health care field has only recently begun to adopt this approach to managing human errors in the medical environment (Leape, 1996). One such effort is the work of the Institute of Healthcare Improvement, which developed a collaborative program among fifty hospitals to learn techniques to eliminate errors in their medication systems in order to reduce adverse events. Techniques ranged from standardized notations for prescriptions (for example, writing out the word "unit" instead of just the letter "u," which can resemble a zero) to redesigning look-alike drug packages and making the packaging of all lethal drugs more distinctive. A fundamental assumption of human factors analysis is that "to err is human" but that improved systems designs can reduce or eliminate the deleterious effects of human errors. In other words, you can't change human nature, but you can change the way a person interacts with the system or the environment in which that individual operates (LaBar, 1996).

From our point of view, an important corollary of this assumption is that humans are more prone to error when they are "under stress, over-worked or subjected to a hostile or punitive environment" (Leape, 1996). Although human factors improvements in medical systems like those described by Leape may not strike at the root causes of stress and burnout among physicians and thus may not seem likely to have much impact on reducing Dr. Weary's stress in the crowded, noisy ER, they do seem likely to reduce the incidence of medical mistakes, a beneficial result that in itself may well have a positive feedback effect on reducing levels of stress among hospital personnel. However, until well-designed studies have been conducted to test this hypothesis, it remains speculative if hopeful. As the Institute of Medicine report shows, however, the time is long overdue for fresh perspectives and new approaches. Systems design innovations in the aerospace and automotive industries can provide useful models for comparable reforms in the health care system. The work of the Institute of Healthcare Improvement described by Leape is a modest but welcome first effort in that direction.

Conclusion

Medical mistakes occur with regularity, and they will always occur. It is a realistic objective, however, to imagine a medical environment in which medical mistakes are far less common than at present. The critical question is how society in general and medicine in particular can achieve this objective. In the past, attention has focused on the track record of the individual health care provider. A physician making a mistake is often sued, competency is questioned, and if the mistake is egregious enough, the individual held at fault may retire, relocate, or otherwise be removed from the medical staff. This process has repeated itself for decades. Unfortunately, without a systematic look at the factors involved and the environment in which a mistake occurs, very little is done to ensure that the replacement provider will not repeat exactly the same process.

One of the global factors that should be evaluated in considering medical error is the stress inherent in today's medical environment. It is our contention that stress affects performance, which in turn produces mistakes. This is a hard contention to prove with data because the important factors are intangible. Who can quantify frustration, inattention, or distraction? And yet no one would argue that the squalling babies in the backseat were not at least partially responsible for the driver's latest fender bender.

Likewise, the abundant sensory inputs provided by new technology, such as the cell phone or GPS navigation devices, may be gradually overwhelming people's ability to process information effectively, with resulting errors in judgment and possibly more than a fender bender as a consequence. If one considers that the driver may also be mentally and physically fatigued before turning the key in the ignition, it is easy to understand how the distracting effects of common stressors would be greatly magnified.

Like the driver of an automobile, the physician is more likely to make a medical mistake when burdened with mental fatigue and environmental stressors. These factors are becoming increasingly important as the pace of modern living accelerates and technological innovation expands. Although it is true that we all face such changes, the consequences are more severe in the medical environment because human lives are so profoundly influenced by medical decision making.

Unfortunately, stress, both mental and environmental, is routinely overlooked as an important systematic cause of medical mistakes. There are direct, easy, and inexpensive ways to reduce stress, particularly in hospitals. It may be hard to make a direct link, but the available evidence and collective common sense suggest that strategies implemented to reduce physician stress will result in fewer medical mistakes.

References

Anderson, J. D., Jay, S. J., Weng, H. C., & Anderson, M. M. (1995). Studying the effect of clinical uncertainty on physicians' decision-making using ILIAD. *MEDINFO*, 8, pt. 2, 869–872.

Brennan, T. A., Leape, L. L., Laird, N. M., Herbert, L., Localio, A. R., Lawthers, A. G., Newhouse, J. P., Weiler, P. C., & Hiatt, H. H. (1991).

Incidence of adverse events and negligence in hospitalized patients: Results of the Harvard Medical Practice Study I. *New England Journal of Medicine, 324,* 370–376.

Campbell, D. A., Jr. (1999). The patient, burnout, and the practice of surgery (Presidential Address). *American Surgeon, 65,* 601–605.

Cohen, S. (1980). Aftereffects of stress on human performance and social behavior: A review of research and theory. *Psychological Bulletin, 88,* 82–108.

Cohen, S., & Spacapan, S. (1978). The aftereffects of stress: An attentional interpretation. *Environmental Psychology and Nonverbal Behavior, 3,* 43–47.

Deary, I. J., & Tait, R. (1987). Effects of sleep disruption on cognitive performance and mood in medical house officers. *British Medical Journal, 295,* 1513–1516.

Deckard, G., Meterko, M., & Field, D. (1994). Physician burnout: An examination of personal, professional, and organizational relationships. *Medical Care, 32,* 745–754.

Dittus, R. S., Roberts, S. D., & Wilson, J. R. (1989). Quantifying uncertainty in medical decisions. *Journal of the American College of Cardiology, 14,* 23A–28A.

Felton, J. S. (1998). Burnout as a clinical entity: Its importance in healthcare workers. *Occupational Medicine, 48,* 237–250.

Firth-Cozens, J. (1993). Stress, psychological problems, and clinical performance. In C. Vincent (Ed.), *Medical accidents* (pp. 131–149). Oxford, UK: Oxford University Press.

Fleger, S. A. (1993, March). Human factors analysis useful for process safety management: Quantitative and qualitative methods help lower frequency, severity of human errors. *Occupational Health and Safety, 4,* 26–27, 30–32.

Hazarding the night [Editorial]. (1994). *Lancet, 344,* 1099–1100.

Jones, J. W. (1988, March). Breaking the vicious stress cycle. *Best's Review,* pp. 74–76.

Jones, J. W., Barge, B. N., Steffy, B. D., Fay, L. M., Kuntz, L. K., & Wuebker, L. J. (1988). Stress and medical malpractice: Organization risk assessment and intervention. *Journal of Applied Psychology, 73,* 727–735.

Kahill, S. (1988). Symptoms of professional burnout: A review of the empirical evidence. *Canadian Psychology, 29,* 284–297.

Kohn, L. T., Corrigan, J. M., & Donaldson, M. S. (Eds.); Committee on Quality of Health Care in America, Institute of Medicine. (2000). *To err is human: Building a safer health system.* Washington, DC: National Academy Press.

Krueger, G. P. (1989). Sustained work, fatigue, sleep loss and performance: A review of the issues. *Work & Stress, 3,* 129–141.

LaBar, G. (1996, April). Can ergonomics cure "human error"? *Occupational Hazards,* pp. 48–51.

Leape, L. L. (1996). Out of the darkness: Hospitals begin to take mistakes seriously. *Health Systems Review, 29,* 21–24.

Leape, L. L., Brennan, T. A., Laird, N. M., Lawthers, A. G., Localio, A. R., Barnes, B. A., Herbert, L. E., Newhouse, J. P., Weiler, P. C., & Hiatt, H. H. (1991). The nature of adverse events in hospitalized patients: Results of the Harvard Medical Practice Study II. *New England Journal of Medicine, 324,* 377–384.

Leiter, M. (1991). The dream denied: Professional burnout and the constraints of human service organizations. *Canadian Psychology, 32,* 547–555.

Maslach, C., & Jackson, S. (1986). *Maslach Burnout Inventory.* Palo Alto, CA: Consulting Psychologists Press.

Meyerson, S. (1990). Under stress? *Practitioner, 234,* 973–976.

Orton, J. I., & Gruzelier, J. H. (1989). Adverse changes in mood and cognitive performance of house officers after night duty. *British Medical Journal, 298,* 21–23.

Pilowski, L., & O'Sullivan, G. (1989). Mental illness in doctors: Common and demands a coordinated response. *British Medical Journal, 298,* 269–270.

Redelmeier, D. A., & Shafir, E. (1995). Medical decision making in situations that offer multiple alternatives. *Journal of the American Medical Association, 273,* 302–305.

Samkoff, J. S., & Jacques, C. H. (1991). A review of studies concerning effects of sleep deprivation and fatigue on residents' performance. *Academic Medicine, 66,* 687–693.

Stern, A., & Keller, R. R. (1991, May). Human error and equipment design in the chemical industry. *Professional Safety,* pp. 37–41.

Svensson, E., Angelborg-Thanderz, M., Sjöberg, L., & Olsson, S. (1997). Information complexity: Mental workload and performance in combat aircraft. *Ergonomics, 40,* 362–380.

Webster, S. (2000, June 25). Ailing hospitals, changing care. *Detroit News,* pp. 1A, 6–7A.

Weinberg, A., & Creed, F. (2000). Stress and psychiatric disorder in healthcare professionals and hospital staff. *Lancet, 355,* 533–537.

3

Medical Error in Primary Care

Michael D. Fetters

The Institute of Medicine (IOM) report *To Err Is Human* synthesizes much of the existing literature on the current state of knowledge about medical errors, the implications for patient safety, and mechanisms to improve safety (Kohn, Corrigan, & Donaldson, 2000). Although previous works have addressed error in surgery and medicine (Bosk, 1979; Bogner, 1994; Rosenthal, Mulcahy, & Lloyd-Bostock, 1999), the IOM report is most significant for having mobilized organized medicine's interest in medical errors and for developing specific policy recommendations for reduction of error and promotion of patient safety. Landmark epidemiological research on adverse events focused attention on errors in hospital settings, and the IOM report highlighted previous studies to demonstrate the need for policies to reduce medical error (Brennan et al., 1991; Leape et al., 1991; Thomas et al., 2000). Though the IOM report convincingly argues the need for policy changes to reduce error in medicine, the report lacks systematic attention to medical errors in primary care practice.

The value of focusing on errors in primary care is compelling because that area's scope includes the specialties of family medicine, general internal medicine, pediatrics, and depending on one's definitions, obstetrics and gynecology. Primary care serves as the portal of entry for most patients in the U.S. health care system, and the vast majority of patient visits occur in the outpatient–primary care setting (White, Williams, & Greenberg, 1961; Green, Fryer, Yawn, Lanier, & Dovey, 2001). Although the bulk of primary care is provided in the outpatient setting, many primary care physicians also provide hospital-based care for general medical problems. Delivering babies and caring for patients in emergency rooms and intensive care units are part of the daily practice of many primary care physicians. Primary care clinicians, who have trained and often continue to practice in both the inpatient and outpatient settings, understand the transitions that affect patients who move between the clinic and the hospital.

Moreover, in the outpatient–primary care setting the most frequent ethical dilemmas encountered are different from those commonly faced in the inpatient–tertiary care setting, the moral agents are systematically different, the setting is different, and even solutions to similar ethical dilemmas often differ (Fetters & Brody, 1999). Investigators of errors in primary care have drawn attention to *behavioral errors*, or *relational errors*, that occur in this setting and how they can result in adverse outcomes that are preventable (Fischer, Fetters, Munro, Goldman, & Goldman, 1997; Fetters & Brody, 1999; Conradi & de Mol, 1999). Moreover, if the recommendations of the IOM report are *not* applied to the primary care context, it will be difficult to illustrate the relevance of medical errors to primary care clinicians and to engage them in efforts to promote patient safety through the reduction of error.

Given the existing research emphasis on errors in inpatient settings and the compelling importance of primary care practice in the U.S. health system, the purpose of this chapter is to review the existing data on medical errors in outpatient–primary care practice and to consider the implications of the IOM report recommendations for the reduction of medical errors in that setting.

What We Know About Medical Errors
in Outpatient–Primary Care Practice

Surprisingly little is known about medical errors in outpatient primary care (Kohn et al., 2000). Previous reports addressing medical errors in primary care practice have examined anecdotal reports of errors (Hilfiker, 1984); family physicians' and generalists' recall of medical errors (Ely, Levinson, Elder, Mainous, & Vinson, 1995; Conradi & de Mol, 1999); the emotional impact of errors (Newman, 1996); generalists' errors in prescribing long-term medications (Britten et al., 1995); patients' preferences for management of medical errors, based on theoretical cases (Witman, Park, & Hardin, 1996); and a series of studies on errors in generalist practice by Dutch physicians (Conradi & de Mol, 1999). Surprisingly, very little research has been conducted on the epidemiology of medical errors in primary care (Fischer et al., 1997; Bhasale, Miller, Reid, & Britt, 1998).

In the only known study conducted to estimate the prevalence of errors in outpatient practice, Fischer et al. (1997) examined the records of a risk management database. The investigators applied the taxonomy used by Brennan et al. (1991) to examine adverse events according to their causes, potential preventability, and outcomes. The prevalence of adverse events was found to be 3.7 per 100,000 clinic visits over five and a half years. Twenty-nine (83 percent) of the thirty-five identified adverse events were attributed to medical errors and considered preventable. Of these twenty-nine, four (14 percent) resulted in permanent disabling injuries, and one (3 percent) resulted in a death. Because the data were obtained from a risk management database primarily designed for malpractice prevention, the identified prevalence is an absolute minimum estimate, and the actual prevalence is most assuredly higher.

A subsequently published study conducted in Australia by 324 general practitioners participating in an incident reporting system examined a total of 805 incidents reported to have occurred from

October 1993 to June 1995 (Bhasale et al., 1998). Of these incidents, 76 percent, a number close to that found by Fischer et al. (1997), were judged preventable, and 27 percent had the potential for severe harm. Unfortunately, the lack of a denominator precluded estimating the incidence of error.

Although not focused on all types of medical errors or necessarily on primary care, the small body of research that has examined medication errors in ambulatory care is also relevant. In one study, 1,000 patient visits to an office-based medical practice were analyzed for adverse drug reactions. These adverse events were identified in 4.2 percent ($n = 42$) of the visits, and slightly more than half of these ($n = 23$) were deemed unnecessary and potentially avoidable (Burnum, 1976). Among 62,216 emergency room visits in a health maintenance organization, Schneitman-McIntire, Farnen, Gordon, Chan, and Toy (1996) found that 1,074 visits (1.7 percent) were attributable to medication noncompliance or mismanagement.

Is Outpatient–Primary Care Practice Safe?

The lack of convincing epidemiological data may, unfortunately, foster a complacent attitude and by default lead to the conclusions that outpatient–primary care practice is very safe for patients, identification and analysis of errors is unnecessary, and little is to be gained through implementation of prevention programs. Such conclusions are problematic.

The opportunities for medical error occurrence in the outpatient–primary care setting are high, and the absolute number of errors may be greater than in the inpatient setting because the vast majority of doctor-patient encounters occur in the outpatient setting (White et al., 1961; Green et al., 2001). Outpatient–primary care practice is growing ever more complex due to the shorter hospitalizations for most illnesses and a concurrent increase in the acuity of illness among patients treated in the outpatient setting—all as appointment slots grow ever shorter under pressure for increased productivity. Previous analyses of outpatient practice have focused on errors of commission, with little attention to errors of omission. Although primary care practice includes many diagnostic and therapeutic interventions, it also has a significant focus on health promotion and disease prevention (primary prevention), early detection (secondary prevention), and minimizing disease progression (tertiary prevention). It has been found that primary care physicians fail to consistently deliver benchmark preventive services; therefore errors of omission are likely to be highly significant. Even well-designed interventions have failed to sustain delivery at targeted levels (Harris, O'Malley, Fletcher, & Knight, 1990; McPhee, Bird, Fordham, Rodnick, & Osborn, 1991; Dietrich, Sox, Tosteson, & Woodruff, 1994; Ruffin, 1998; Hillman et al., 1998; U.S. Department of Health and Human Services, Public Health Service, 1999).

Reduction of medical errors in primary care could yield far greater margins of improvement in health than reduction of error in hospital-based systems alone. Among physicians, primary care specialists take the brunt of responsibility for attacking the most common actual causes of death, namely, tobacco, diet and activity patterns, alcohol, microbial agents, toxic agents, firearms, sexual behavior, motor vehicles, and illicit drug use (McGinnis & Foege, 1993). Primary care physicians' presence in and contributions to the community could translate into enhanced opportunities to develop the community-based collaborative initiatives envisioned in the IOM report. Unfortunately, demonstrating the benefits of preventive interventions in reducing deaths from these common root causes may prove difficult because the result of intervening may not be noticed until years or decades after the interventions begin. Although the Australian incident monitoring study collected various errors recognized by the reporting general practitioners, these were largely errors of commission (Bhasale et al., 1998). Creative efforts to document the errors of omission and their overall impact are greatly needed.

In short the existing studies and the analysis offered here illustrate that medical errors occur in outpatient–primary care practice, many of them are preventable, and standard risk management reporting systems that rely on voluntary filing of *incident reports* in the context of a system still eager to find a bad apple are ineffective. Outpatient–primary care practice cannot be assumed to be safe due to the many opportunities for error. Given the importance of errors in primary care and the role primary care physicians can play in their reduction, there is a need to assess the implications of the Institute of Medicine report for this setting.

IOM Recommendations and Their Implications for Primary Care

The IOM Committee on Quality of Health Care in America laid out a series of recommendations for patient safety and overall quality and created a national agenda for reducing errors in health care and improving patient safety (Kohn et al., 2000, Executive Summary). The report made recommendations in four areas: developing leadership and knowledge, identifying and learning from errors, raising standards and expectations for improvement, and creating safety systems inside health care organizations. How do these recommendations apply to primary care?

Developing Leadership and Knowledge

To develop the leadership, research, tools, and protocols to enhance our knowledge base about safety, recommendation 4.1 of the IOM report calls for the creation of a Center for Patient Safety. As illustrated previously, primary care practice differs greatly from hospital-based care in terms of the types of problems seen, the systems used in the delivery of care, and the practice environment itself. Primary care physicians' active participation in both outpatient and inpatient care gives them a comprehensive view of the implications of policy changes. They can contribute a unique perspective on how particular policies or recommendations would affect both inpatient and outpatient care, as well as on how to implement these recommendations in patient transitions from outpatient to inpatient to outpatient settings. Primary care physician representation will be needed in efforts to identify the research agenda, investigate the nature of errors in primary care, and design interventions to reduce error in primary care.

Identifying and Learning from Errors

To identify and learn from errors, the IOM report argues for a nationwide, mandatory reporting system. Recommendation 5.1 calls for standardized collection of information about adverse events that result in death or serious harm. As previous studies on errors in primary care have revealed, developing systems for accurately detecting events and determining the frequency with which they occur, particularly for errors of omission, has proven difficult (Fischer et al., 1997; Bhasale et al., 1998). Recommendation 5.2 calls for the development of voluntary reporting efforts. However, the unique practice environment and the heterogeneity of practice systems and organization in primary care must be considered when such systems are developed.

Recommendation 6.1 calls for legislation to extend peer review protections to data related to patient safety and quality improvement. Although primary care physicians experience less malpractice litigation than physicians in many other specialties do, they are nonetheless anxious about public disclosure of error and the potential for litigation (Goold, Hofer, Zimmerman, & Hayward, 1994; Breslin, Taylor, & Brodsky, 1986; Shapiro et al., 1989). This derives in part from the perpetuation of the bad-apple theory of medical errors by physicians and the failure to recognize health care as a system (Van Cott, 1994; Moray, 1994). Data collection systems and the content of those systems must be primary care friendly and developed with the input of the clinicians who will be affected by the reporting systems. Participation by primary care practitioners is essential for developing appropriate outcome measures and the nomenclature and taxonomy needed to facilitate reporting. Experience suggests that practice-based research networks have the potential to be translated into viable voluntary systems for reporting on adverse events (Nutting, Beasley, & Werner, 1999).

Setting Performance Standards and Expectations for Safety

IOM recommendation 7.1 calls for health care organizations to focus greater attention on safety. The IOM suggests public and private health care purchasers use three tools to demand attention to safety: (1) considering patient safety in contracting decisions, (2) providing information about clinicians' safety practices to employees or beneficiaries, and (3) conveying concerns about safety to accrediting bodies. Safety practice benchmarks developed in collaboration with primary care physicians will result in measures that are both relevant to and feasible within the clinical context of outpatient practice. Primary care physicians' input can help guide efforts to promote a cultural environment that is not punitive.

Recommendation 7.2 calls for health professionals' performance standards and expectations to focus more on patient safety. Many primary care organizations could help develop procedures for assessing practitioners' competence and knowledge about safety practices and develop educational opportunities to correct identified deficiencies. Development of curricula on patient safety could be coordinated among such organizations as the American Academy of Family Physicians, the Society of Teachers of Family Medicine, the North American Primary Care Research Group, the Society of General Internal Medicine, and the American Academy of Pediatrics.

Dissemination of information about advances in patient safety could be coordinated through entities such as the *Journal of the American Board of Family Practice*, the American Board of Internal Medicine, the *American Family Physician*, the *Journal of Family Practice*, the *Journal of General Internal Medicine*, and so forth. To formulate patient safety considerations as guidelines, as suggested by the IOM report, will require a clear understanding of the most common and potentially serious errors that occur in primary care practice. Collaboration at national summits among the diverse disciplines represented by these organizations and publications may require creation of scholarships or incentives to promote cross-fertilization in specialty meetings, which currently tend *not* to be interdisciplinary.

IOM recommendation 7.3 suggests that the Food and Drug Administration (FDA) increase attention to the safe use of drugs and that it collaborate with physicians and pharmacists to establish appropriate responses to problems identified through postmarketing surveillance. Primary care physicians' roles in prescribing a large variety of medications, dispensing medications (in some settings), and monitoring patient response to treatment position them to assist the FDA in unique ways.

Implementing Safety Systems in Health Care

The specific recommendations of the IOM report on the implementation of safety systems in health care are deceptively brief, but the possible ways to achieve them are enormously rich. Recommendation 8.1 calls for health care organizations and professionals to make patient safety a declared and serious aim with defined executive responsibility. In contrast to complex social institutions such as hospitals and health maintenance organizations, where changes are difficult to achieve, private practitioners do have significant control over operations in their practices. This means that outpatient–primary care practitioners have many opportunities to follow the IOM recommendations for implementing safety. For example, they can (1) take a leadership role in focusing attention on safety in their practice settings, (2) implement nonpunitive systems for reporting and analyzing errors within their organizations, (3) incorporate safety principles into their practices, and (4) initiate team training programs such as simulations to enhance patient safety in their practices.

At the same time, it will be difficult to find leadership accountable to and esteemed by the nation's heterogeneous groups of internists, family physicians, pediatricians, general practitioners (generalists not certified in a specialty), and others who consider themselves primary care physicians. One current effort (Genetics in Primary Care: A Faculty Development Initiative) may provide a model for such interdisciplinary collaboration (Binder, 1998).

The IOM report proposed five principles for the design of safety systems. They are outlined in Table 3.1; issues of particular relevance to primary care physicians are highlighted in the third and fourth columns.

Some of the difficulties of implementing the IOM recommendations are outlined in the report itself (Kohn et al., 2000, p. 167). For example, the report emphasizes that community-based physicians need to develop a sense of belonging to organized structures such as hospitals, managed care organizations, medical societies, medical practice groups, and so forth.

There are additional significant barriers not mentioned in Table 3.1. Not the least of these are financial constraints. Most ambulatory primary care practices are streamlined, with tightly controlled budgets and personnel. The ratcheting down of reimbursement for medical services has now made staffing even tighter. In this context, it will be difficult to spend more time and money on safety unless policies with financial incentives (or, less desirably, penalties) are adopted. Given these financial constraints, the safety programs implemented are likely to rely on greater vigilance, a phenomenon the report specifically recommends against. Although vigilance is presumed to be a good quality in doctors, it is not a robust system for error detection and prevention. All the suggested principles involve significant costs in time and effort.

There may be cultural barriers to implementation as well. Many community-based primary care practitioners have an entrepreneurial spirit and may find many of the egalitarian notions of responsibilities and relationships proposed by the IOM to be unacceptable.

Table 3.1. Principles for the Design of Safety Systems in Health Care Organizations.

Principle	Processes	Relevance for Outpatient Primary Care	Barriers to Implementation in Outpatient Care
1. Provide leadership.	Make patient safety a priority corporate objective.	Easier to do in smaller outpatient practices because of less organizational complexity.	Difficult to emphasize in a for-profit practice because changes perceived as costly.
	Make patient safety everyone's responsibility.	Feasible but dependent on incorporating safety into the practice philosophy.	Most practices and staff are already stretched thin, and there are no incremental rewards for doing more work.
	Make clear assignments for and expectations of safety oversight.	Same as above; also, increased accountability requires reducing other commitments.	Making assignments is easy, but leadership and follow-up require physician commitment.
	Provide human and financial resources for error analysis and systems redesign.	Need to develop a reward system such as a special accreditation system as a selling point for practices to meet the standards.	May be perceived as elitist by nonparticipating physicians; resources have to come from practicing physicians with limited resources and staff.

2. Respect human limits in process design.	Develop effective mechanisms for dealing with unsafe practitioners.	Given historical trends, primary care physicians seem unlikely to accept such mechanisms without several cases handled well.	Practitioners uncomfortable with reporting colleagues and with being "whistle-blowers."
	Design jobs for safety.	Highly relevant for nursing staff and physicians.	Lack of expertise in minimizing risk in health occupations.
	Avoid reliance on memory.	Need greater use of table-top, palm-top, and other types of electronic technology.	Must change current practice pattern of overreliance on memory in clinical care.
	Use constraints and forcing functions (using parameters and interventions to limit errors).	Many already in place, but can develop further.	Must change the status quo.
	Avoid reliance on vigilance.	The response to efforts to improve safety will likely be a call for greater vigilance.	Default pattern for "doing more" is in fact increased vigilance.

(continued)

Table 3.1. Principles for the Design of Safety Systems in Health Care Organizations (*continued*).

Principle	Processes	Relevance for Outpatient Primary Care	Barriers to Implementation in Outpatient Care
	Simplify key processes.	Necessary and may achieve other savings for practitioners.	Tendency to maintain the status quo; requires resources to develop.
	Standardize work processes.	May reap additional benefits in terms of increased efficiency.	Same as above.
3. Promote effective team functioning.	Train in teams those expected to work in teams.	Local control of practices makes implementation easier.	In smaller offices the same people will be involved in all efforts.
	Include the patient in safety and design efforts.	Likely to be informative.	Involving patients may be uncomfortable for providers.
4. Anticipate the unexpected.	Adopt a proactive approach: examine processes of care for threats to safety and redesign them before accidents occur.	Requires identification of the most important threats to patient safety.	Creating time and resources to examine and redesign.

5. Create a learning environment.	Design for recovery.	Same as above.	Same as above.
	Improve access to accurate, timely information.	Same as above.	Incidents may be so infrequent that interest atrophies.
	Use simulations whenever possible.	Likely to be highly effective and valuable for practices not already doing so.	Requires contemplating the threats to safety and developing simulations.
	Encourage reporting of errors and hazardous conditions.	Requires recognition of the most important issues and development of monitoring systems.	Environment of blame pervades; perception of legal culpability remains.
	Ensure no reprisals for reporting of errors.	Dependent on leadership in the offices and the organization.	More difficult in small settings, where everybody knows everyone and a "boss" may be central to the etiology.
	Develop a working culture in which communication flows freely regardless of authority gradient.	Practice structures and cultures are highly variable.	Private practitioners by nature may be authoritarian and resistant to notions of equality.
	Implement mechanisms of feedback and learning from error.	Requires overcoming structures of authority.	Requires resources and change in culture.

Also, because these practitioners may feel particular resistance toward changes they feel have been developed with an eye toward hospital-based care, systems organized to promote collaboration with other ambulatory care entities rather than with hospitals may make most sense. Overcoming the status quo will require the leadership of the previously mentioned primary care specialty groups, especially in the creation of an effective learning environment for such historically independent and entrepreneurial practitioners. Such groups could be instrumental in development of continuing medical education modules — similar to Advanced Life Support in Obstetrics (ALSO), Neonatal Resuscitation Program (NRP), and Advanced Cardiac Life Support (ACLS)—that address problems encountered by primary care practitioners. These organizations can also support the development of appropriate medical error taxonomies and of monitoring and reporting systems.

Recommendation 8.2 urges health care organizations to implement proven medication safety practices, and most of the recommendations are straightforward, as illustrated in the following list.

Selected Strategies to Improve Medication Safety

1. Adopt a system-oriented approach to medication error reduction.

2. Implement standard processes for medication doses, dose time, and dose scales in a given patient care unit.

3. Standardize prescription writing and prescribing rules.

4. Limit the number of different kinds of common equipment.

5. Implement physician order entry.

6. Use pharmaceutical software.

7. Implement unit dosing.

8. Have a central pharmacy supply high-risk medications.

9. Use special procedures and written protocols for high-risk medications.

10. Do not store concentrated solutions of hazardous medications on patient care units.

11. Ensure the availability of pharmaceutical decision support.

12. Include a pharmacist during rounds on patient care units.

13. Make relevant patient information available at the point of patient care.

14. Improve patients' knowledge about their treatment.

The overarching strategy is to adopt a systems-oriented approach to medication error reduction. Primary care physicians already follow many of these suggested practices and can readily build on them. Standardizing processes to minimize complexity stands as the most important practice. Points that are particularly relevant to outpatient–primary care practitioners include the need for greater care in writing prescriptions and the potential power of using computer-based programs for examining drug interactions. Several Japanese patients entering my practice have brought from Japan a patient education sheet for medication, with the drug name and a color picture of the drug and information about dosage and timing, drug purpose, and potential common or dangerous side effects. The technology for such interventions is clearly available but needs to be applied and disseminated.

Implementing Error Prevention Systems in Primary Care

There is a growing call to draw from systems theory to reduce medical errors, and there is good reason to believe such a systems approach offers great promise for reduction of medical errors in primary care. It is unclear, however, which approaches will be the most effective. Leape et al. (1995) have highlighted the aviation model's systems approach to error reduction, a model that has been successfully applied to reduction of medical errors. Unfortunately, the aviation model of error reduction may not translate nearly as well for primary care as it has for repetitive hospital-based services such as anesthesia.

In primary care, clinicians deal with an enormous range of illnesses and medical problems (Stange et al., 1998). In a given day, a practitioner might not see a particular clinical problem more than once. Family physicians and many other primary care physicians also see a broad range of patients of various ages. For the same presenting complaint, the diagnostic workup and treatment course for various patients might differ dramatically. For example, workup and management of a geriatric man, a twenty-five-year-old woman, and a child, all with lower abdominal pain, can be very different because the most likely etiologies are dependent on the patient's age and the history of present illness.

Moreover, ambulatory patients vary considerably in their compliance with a recommended regimen. In the outpatient setting, compliance with a recommended regimen for treating diabetes mellitus is highly dependent upon the patient. In contrast, a hospitalized diabetic patient receives medication at regularly scheduled times each day, and a nurse watches to see that the medication is actually taken.

Finally, geographical considerations affect systems implementation. Hospitals consolidate a large number of patients into one geographical setting where hundreds of doctors can collaborate through existing computers and support systems. Although the number of solo practices has decreased, many primary care physicians still conduct their clinical practices in small-group settings in the community. The office systems used in these diverse practices vary enormously. Office staff with similar titles may perform quite different functions in different settings. The systems implemented in primary care will need to be highly versatile and user friendly and must account for the complex behavioral and cognitive processes that recur in primary care if they are to be effective (Conradi & de Mol, 1999).

Conclusion

The analysis in this chapter delineates the magnitude of the agenda for research on medical errors in primary care. Development and testing of a taxonomy that reflects the nature of outpatient–primary care practice is the most compelling item on that agenda for realizing the goal of reducing error and promoting patient safety in this setting. It will be highly difficult to find, count, and prevent errors in primary care when there is no agreement on what qualifies. An effective taxonomy should include types of errors and their etiologies, and as illustrated in Table 3.2, it could also include specific examples from primary care for clarification.

Upon the development of a taxonomy of errors appropriate for primary care, more sophisticated research on the epidemiology should be conducted as previous research is inadequate due to incomplete data for the numerator (Fischer et al., 1997) or the denominator (Bhasale et al., 1998) or due to a narrow focus on a specific type of error (Schneitman-McIntire et al., 1996). With this epidemiological data, it will be possible to develop priorities for error prevention and design the interventions necessary to make primary care practice safer.

A more thorough examination and discussion of the ethical and legal issues associated with medical errors and of the recommendations for conveying information about discovered errors should proceed in parallel with the research efforts previously described. Physicians need a clear understanding of the legal and ethical implications of error monitoring and disclosure. Although some authors argue in favor of full, routine disclosure of errors (Peterson & Brennan, 1990; Fetters, 1995; Foubister, 2000), some risk management authorities argue against disclosure to the patient unless there

Table 3.2. Taxonomy of Etiologies of Medical Errors.

Etiologies	Manifestations and Clinical Examples
Deficient knowledge	• Never learned a particular entity (physician cannot recognize scleroderma) • Failure to update knowledge (patient not started on beta blocker after myocardial infarction) • Failure to obtain adequate history from the patient (previous attempted suicide events not elicited) • Relevant physical findings not found because omitted from physical examination (friction rub of pericardial effusion not detected) • Failure to recognize specific physical findings (squamous cell carcinoma)
Deficient judgment or cognitive skills	• Misdiagnosis of one disease entity for another (appendicitis misdiagnosed as gastroenteritis) • Failure to develop and consider differential diagnosis (pulmonary embolism in patient with atypical chest pain; neurosyphilis in elderly patient with memory loss) • Failure to recognize own limits in ability to identify and/or treat the patient • Failure to obtain second opinion • Failure to schedule follow-up (cellulitis progresses) • Ineffective treatment plan for properly diagnosed illness
Deficient psycho-motor skills	• Infrequent performance of a particular procedure (flexible sigmoidoscopy) • Technically deficient performance of a physical examination skill (fundoscopic examination, Barany maneuvers, mental status evaluation)

Etiologies	Manifestations and Clinical Examples
Internal systems failure	• Equipment malfunction (can be unavoidable or avoidable, if for example no attention to maintenance) • Necessary item for procedure either not stocked or insufficiently stocked (culture media for Group B streptococcus of pregnancy; EKG paper)
External systems failure	• Computerized database entry system too complex (cumbersome immunization database or prenatal care information) • Computer system crashes • "Production quotas" set that strain medical staff availability for practice of medicine • Frequent changes in guidelines (changes in recommendations for rotavirus, elimination of thimerosol-containing vaccines and subsequent availability of mixed vaccines [Hib and Hep B])
Inadequate staffing	• Insufficient cleaning or sterilization of instruments (sigmoidoscope, speculums) • Inattention to procedure or patient care • Too few staff to assist with procedures
Poor documentation	• Dictation system failure, dead batteries, worn-out or broken equipment • Failure of staff to deliver dictation tapes • Failure of physician to dictate in complete or timely fashion (recall error including omission of data or inaccurate description)
Inadequate or inaccurate data	• Medical history incompletely elicited by the physician • Medical history inaccurately reported by the patient (intentionally or unintentionally) • Relevant medical history not reported by the patient • Medical record not available

(continued)

Table 3.2. Taxonomy of Etiologies of Medical Errors (*continued*).

Etiologies	Manifestations and Clinical Examples
	• Laboratory data turnaround is too long (INR performed on Friday not available over holiday weekend until Tuesday)
	• Scheduling of testing delayed due to long wait times (delay for mammogram)
Improper supervision	• Nurse practitioner or resident lacks technical skills and fails to ask for supervision
	• Nurse practitioner or resident asks for assistance that is not received
	• Supervising physician not accessible when needed by subordinate
	• Inadequately trained medical staff
Inadequate follow-up	• Patient misses appointment
	• Physician doesn't schedule patient follow-up
Failure to integrate prevention	• Pneumovax or tetanus vaccine not provided; failure to counsel smoking cessation, osteoporosis prevention
Miscommunication	• Verbal order confused due to similarity of names (HiB given rather than Hep B vaccine)
	• Verbal order communicated ambiguously (patient gets peak flows instead of spirometry due to verbal order for "lung function testing")
	• Miscommunication with a covering physician or consultant about patient management (failure to mention patient's DNR status, family or patient preferences for management)
Failure to communicate	• Abnormal diagnostic test not conveyed in timely way to patient (mammogram, hemoccult)
	• Abnormal diagnostic test never conveyed to patient
Failure to convey empathy	• Poor patient compliance with follow-up and treatment recommendations (cerebrovascular accident secondary to uncontrolled hypertension)

Etiologies	Manifestations and Clinical Examples
Time pressures	• Busy schedule prevents physician from adequate attention to a specific clinical problem (failure to identify patient with suicidal thoughts)
Cavalier personality	• Overconfidence in technical skills (performs new procedure without previous experience, or performs familiar procedure in atypical circumstances)

was injury (Tennenhouse & Kasher, 1988). Although there appears to be a trend for hospital risk managers to disclose errors, corporate groups may be less financially vulnerable, due to their size, than a private practitioner or group practice in the outpatient setting (Prager, 1998). Some states have enacted laws that protect *benevolent gestures* such as an apology from being admitted as evidence in a malpractice case. Such measures are helpful, though physicians will likely still feel vulnerable, because distinguishing between expressing sorrow and admitting fault is difficult (Prager, 1998). Primary care physicians who develop close relationships with patients and communities and provide continuous care over time rather than episodic care may feel particularly vulnerable.

The barriers to achieving the IOM goals of patient safety in the outpatient–primary care setting can be overcome but are significant. Although the approaches and systems developed in inpatient settings are applicable, the unique features of the outpatient–primary care environment and its practitioners must be considered in order to maximize safety. The unique role primary care practitioners play in the overall health system positions them to make especially substantive contributions to safety owing to their opportunities for reducing errors of omission through improvements in health promotion and disease prevention, for testing new systems in less complex environments, and for facilitating seamless approaches to safety in patient transitions between the outpatient and inpatient settings.

References

Bhasale, A. L., Miller, G. C., Reid, S. E., & Britt, H. C. (1998). Analyzing potential harm in Australian general practice: An incident-monitoring study. *Medical Journal of Australia, 169,* 73–76.

Binder, P. (1998, November). Results of human genome research will challenge, help FPs. *FP Report,* pp. 1, 4.

Bogner, M. S. (Ed.). (1994). *Human error in medicine.* Mahway, NJ: Erlbaum.

Bosk, C. (1979). *Forgive and remember: Managing medical failure.* Chicago: University of Chicago Press.

Brennan, T. A., Leape, L. L., Laird, N. M., Herbert, L. E., Localio, A. R., Lawthers, A. G., Newhouse, J. P., Weiler, P. C., & Hiatt, H. H. (1991). Incidence of adverse events and negligence in hospitalized patients: Results of the Harvard Medical Practice Study I. *New England Journal of Medicine, 324,* 370–376.

Breslin, F. A., Taylor, K. R., & Brodsky, S. L. (1986). Development of a litigaphobia scale: Measurement of excessive fear of litigation. *Psychological Reports, 58,* 547–550.

Britten, N., Brant, S., Cairns, A., Jones, I., Salisbury, C., Virji, A., & Herxheimer, A. (1995). Continued prescribing of inappropriate drugs in general practice. *Journal of Clinical Pharmacy and Therapeutics, 20,* 199–205.

Burnum, J. F. (1976). Preventability of adverse drug reactions. *Annals of Internal Medicine, 85,* 80–81.

Conradi, M. H., & de Mol, B.A.J.M. (1999). Research on errors and safety in Dutch general and hospital practice. In M. M. Rosenthal, L. Mulcahy, & S. Lloyd-Bostock (Eds.), *Medical mishaps: Pieces of the puzzle* (pp. 74–83). Bristol, PA: Open University Press.

Dietrich, A., Sox, C. H., Tosteson, T. D., & Woodruff, C. B. (1994). Durability of improved physician early detection of cancer after conclusion of intervention support. *Cancer Epidemiology, Biomarkers & Prevention, 3,* 335–340.

Ely, J. W., Levinson, W., Elder, N. C., Mainous, A. G., III, & Vinson, D. C. (1995). Perceived causes of family physicians' errors. *Journal of Family Practice, 40,* 337–344.

Fetters, M. D. (1995). Error in medicine [Commentary]. *Journal of the American Medical Association, 274,* 458.

Fetters, M. D., & Brody, H. (1999). The epidemiology of bioethics. *Journal of Clinical Ethics, 10,* 107–115.

Fischer, G., Fetters, M. D., Munro, A. P., Goldman, E. B., & Goldman, J. D. (1997). Adverse events in primary care identified from a risk management database. *Journal of Family Practice, 45*, 40–46.

Foubister, V. (2000, August). Broadening the role of forgiveness in medicine. *American Medical News, 21*, 9, 15.

Goold, S. D., Hofer, T., Zimmerman, M., & Hayward, R. A. (1994). Measuring physician attitudes toward cost, uncertainty, malpractice and utilization review. *Journal of General Internal Medicine, 9*, 544–549.

Green, L. A., Fryer, G. E., Jr., Yawn, B. P., Lanier, D., & Dovey, S. M. (2001). The ecology of medical care revisited. *New England Journal of Medicine, 344*, 2021–2025.

Harris, R. P., O'Malley, M. S., Fletcher, S. W., & Knight, B. P. (1990). Prompting physicians for preventive procedures: A five-year study of manual and computer reminders. *American Journal of Preventive Medicine, 6*, 145–152.

Hilfiker, D. (1984). Sounding board: Facing our mistakes. *New England Journal of Medicine, 310*, 118–122.

Hillman, A. L., Ripley, K., Goldfarb, N., Nuamah, I., Weiner, J., & Lusk, E. (1998). Physician financial incentives and feedback: Failure to increase cancer screening in Medicaid managed care. *American Journal of Public Health, 88*, 1699–1701.

Kohn, L. T. (2000). To err is human: An interview with the Institute of Medicine's Linda Kohn. *Joint Commission Journal of Quality Improvement, 26*, 227–234.

Kohn, L. T., Corrigan, J. M., & Donaldson, M. S. (Eds.); Committee on Quality of Health Care in America, Institute of Medicine. (2000). *To err is human: Building a safer health system.* Washington, DC: National Academy Press.

Leape, L. L., Bates, D. W., Cullen, D. J., Cooper, J., Demonaco, H. J., Gallivan, T., Hallisey, R., Ives, J., Laird, N., Laffel, G., Nemeskal, R., Petersen, L. A., Porter, K., Servi, D., Shea, B. F., Small, S. D., Sweitzer, B. J., Thompson, B. T., & Vander Vliet, M. (1995). Systems analysis of adverse drug events. *Journal of the American Medical Association, 274*, 35–43.

Leape, L. L., Brennan, T. A., Laird, N. M., Lawthers, A. G., Localio, A. R., Barnes, B. A., Herbert, L. E., Newhouse, J. P., Weiler, P. C., & Hiatt, H. H. (1991). The nature of adverse events in hospitalized patients: Results of the Harvard Medical Practice Study II. *New England Journal of Medicine, 324*, 377–384.

McGinnis, J. M., & Foege, W. H. (1993). Actual causes of death in the United States. *Journal of the American Medical Association, 270*, 2207–2212.

McPhee, S. J., Bird, J. A., Fordham, D., Rodnick, J. E., & Osborn, E. H. (1991). Promoting cancer prevention activities by primary care physicians. *Journal of the American Medical Association, 266*, 538–544.

Moray, N. (1994). Error reduction as a systems problem. In M. S. Bogner (Ed.), *Human error in medicine* (pp. 67–91). Mahway, NJ: Erlbaum.

Newman, M. C. (1996). The emotional impact of mistakes on family physicians. *Archives of Family Medicine, 5*, 71–75.

Nutting, P. A., Beasley, J. W., & Werner, J. J. (1999). Practice-based research networks answer primary care questions. *Journal of the American Medical Association, 281*, 686–688.

Peterson, L. M., & Brennan, T. A. (1990). Medical ethics and medical injuries: Taking our duties seriously. *Journal of Clinical Ethics, 1*, 207–211.

Prager, L. O. (1998, August). New laws let doctors say "I'm sorry." *American Medical News, 21*, 9, 14, 16.

Rosenthal, M. M., Mulcahy, L., & Lloyd-Bostock, S. (Eds.). (1999). *Medical mishaps: Pieces of the puzzle.* Bristol, PA: Open University Press.

Ruffin, M. T. (1998). Can we change physicians' practices in the delivery of cancer-preventive services? *Archives of Family Medicine, 7*, 317–319.

Schneitman-McIntire, O., Farnen, T. A., Gordon, N., Chan, J., & Toy, W. A. (1996). Medication misadventures resulting in emergency department visits at an HMO medical center. *American Journal of Health-System Pharmacy, 3*, 1416–1422.

Shapiro, R. S., Simpson, D. E., Lawrence, S. L., Talsky, A. M., Sobocinski, K. A., & Schiedermayer, D. L. (1989). A survey of sued and nonsued physicians and suing patients. *Archives of Internal Medicine, 149*, 2190–2196.

Stange, K. C., Zyzanski, S. J., Flocke, S. A., Kelly, R., Jaén, C. R., Miller, W. L., Crabtree, B. F., Callahan, E. J., Gillanders, W. R., Shank, J. C., Chao, J., Medalie, J. H., Gilchrist, V., Goodwin, M. A., & Langa, D. M. (1998). Illuminating the "black box": A description of 4454 patient visits to 138 family physicians. *Journal of Family Practice, 46*, 377–389.

Tennenhouse, D. J., & Kasher, M. P. (1988). *Risk prevention skills: Communicating and record keeping in clinical practice.* San Rafael, CA: Tennenhouse.

Thomas, E. J., Studdert, D. M., Burstin, H. R., Orav, J., Zeena, T., Williams, E. J., Howard, K. M., Weiler, P. C., & Brennan, T. A. (2000). Incidence and types of adverse events and negligent care in Utah and Colorado. *Medical Care, 38*, 261–271.

U.S. Department of Health and Human Services, Public Health Service. (1999). *Healthy People 2000: National health promotion and disease prevention objectives.* Rockville, MD: Author.

Van Cott, H. (1994). Human errors: Their causes and reduction. In M. S. Bogner (Ed.), *Human error in medicine* (pp. 53–65). Mahway, NJ: Erlbaum.

White, K. L., Williams, T. F., & Greenberg, B. G. (1961). The ecology of medical care. *New England Journal of Medicine, 265,* 885–892.

Witman, A. B., Park, D. M., & Hardin, S. B. (1996). How do patients want
physicians to handle mistakes? A survey of internal medicine patients in
an academic setting. *Archives of Internal Medicine, 156,* 2565–2569.

4

Nurses and the "Code of Silence"

Beverly Jones

I ntolerance with medical mishaps has a long legacy. The expectation of flawless performance from physicians can be traced back to the beginning of civilization. The code of Hammurabi, drafted more than a thousand years before the Hippocratic oath, held surgeons accountable for mishaps, threatening the loss of a forehand if they caused death or blindness to a patient (Orlikoff & Vanagunas, 1988). The sense that individual blame and punishment should be apportioned for medical mishaps has expanded over time to include nonphysicians, such as nurses, and entire health care institutions as well.

History, aided by what appears to be an even more narrow societal view, has perpetuated the unrealistic expectation of clinical perfection. Recent medical mistakes have initiated a range of reactions, many of which have been devastatingly punitive and humiliating. Consider the following two examples.

In 1997, in Colorado, three nurses were indicted on charges of negligent homicide following a medication error in a Denver-area hospital that resulted in the death of a newborn infant. In January 1998, two of the nurses pleaded guilty in response to a plea bargain offered by the district attorney's office. The third nurse, who refused the plea bargain, was acquitted. The Institute for Safe Medication Practices performed an in-depth system analysis of the error in this latter case, identifying over fifty different system failures that allowed the error to occur. The institute's work informed the perspectives of the members of the jury and emphasized the importance of looking beyond the idea of blaming a specific person to the greater need for system reform. This analysis also acknowledged the importance of taking a systems approach as a critical step in reform of a system in which mistakes occur (Smetzer, 1998).

The second example involves the Massachusetts State Board of Registration in Nursing (BORN), which proposed sanctions against eighteen nurses who cared for two patients over the course of four days. It was discovered two months later that the two patients had received four times the intended amount of a high-dose chemotherapy. Both patients suffered cardiac injury, and one died. The overdoses were reported around the world and raised many questions. The Massachusetts Department of Public Health, the Joint Commission on Accreditation of Healthcare Organizations (JCAHO), a Dana-Farber Cancer Institute internal investigation, and the National Institutes of Health all found no fault with any of the individual nurses. Four years after the overdoses occurred, BORN proposed licensure sanctions against the nurses, without having conducted an investigation or having any direct dialogue with the nurses. This unfortunate experience was also shared with the entire world. The incident raised public awareness and called attention to the need to monitor the quality of care for patients everywhere (Grant, 1999).

This chapter examines the imperatives for establishing systems that help institutions and individuals avoid medical error and analyzes the barriers that continue to stand in the way of system implementation. It focuses particularly on the barriers embedded in individuals' beliefs about their roles, professional cultural values, and organizational culture that act to discourage individuals, especially physicians and nurses, from collaborating freely in shaping an organizational culture that firmly supports systems that identify and reduce medical mishaps.

The Myth of Perfect Performance

Health care professionals, including physicians and nurses, are socialized to believe that perfect performance is an attainable goal
and that mistakes are due primarily to inattentiveness and care-
lessness. Banister, Butt, & Hackel (1996), discussing "how nurses
perceive medication errors," state that nurses believe good nurses
do not make medication errors. JCAHO (1998) makes the point
that medical and nursing schools reinforce the concept of precision
by discussing the smallest details of cases and illustrating associated
decisions in a manner that makes the outcomes seem obvious. Students are led to conclude that mistakes are not expected to occur
and perfection is attainable. This attitude, coupled with the various punishments meted out for errors (receiving a failing grade, re-
peating a class, or being talked about by peers and instructors),
establishes indelible impressions of fear.

Precision is not only taught in professional educational programs,
it is also reinforced in the health care settings that employ nurses
and physicians. On the one hand, although most medical mishaps
are the subject of hushed hallway gossip, until recently medical
mishaps by physicians have seldom been openly discussed. On the
other hand, mishaps by nurses and other staff are handled much
more publicly, as the two cases cited earlier clearly demonstrate.

Requiring a high standard of performance for health care providers is both appropriate and highly desirable. However, emphasizing this kind of standard as a norm can create a doubled-edged,
psychological sword. It can indeed reinforce a sense of responsibility, yet it may also reinforce the pressure to cover up mistakes (Leape,
1994). As Moore (1999) points out in an assessment of an operating room, commitment to perfection and zero tolerance for mistakes
in a health care setting are reassuring goals in many ways. However, if mistakes are not strategically managed by acknowledging
human vulnerabilities along with systems issues, the individuals
involved may develop poor interpersonal relationships and an un-

willingness to accept accountability. Such attitudes, paradoxically, can foster an environment in which the risk of error is increased.

Recent Efforts to Improve Safety

The release of the Institute of Medicine report on medical errors, *To Err Is Human* (Kohn, Corrigan, & Donaldson, 2000), has brought unprecedented responses from health care organizations and other interested stakeholders. This overwhelming attention is long overdue and heartening. The pioneering efforts of several well-known institutions are establishing sound models for others to emulate (see, for example, Leape, 2000; Paul, 2000; Rebillot, 2000; Reese, 2000).

Stimulated by the untimely death of two of its patients, the Dana-Farber Cancer Institute has pioneered new systems to prevent mistakes in the delivery of chemotherapy agents. The institute has established a computerized system for medication orders, implemented efforts to strengthen care delivery, and is endeavoring to create an institutional culture that encourages the reporting of errors. A new patient-family advisory council advises staff on ways to enhance care, and council members may accompany the medical staff on hospital rounds. A dramatic increase in staff reporting of errors and near misses is one result of these new approaches.

Luther-Midelfort Hospital, part of the Mayo Regional Health System, has also experienced rewarding results from its reform initiatives. Roger Resar, M.D., taking on the charge to reduce medication errors, has centered Luther-Midelfort's efforts on improving the technical aspects of the error reporting process and increasing patient safety at specific points of care. For example, improving medication information gathering by nurses during the admitting process and pharmacy involvement in the discharge medication process has contributed to an 82 percent decrease in medication errors.

At Fairview Health Services, a system of seven hospitals in Minneapolis, the pharmacy was selected to lead the reform efforts.

Fairview's strategies have centered around improving processes and structures so that it is difficult for workers to make mistakes. One of these initiatives, the assignment of pharmacists as case managers for cardiology patients receiving warfarin, has reduced the complication rate for bleeding from 12 percent to 2 percent.

All these efforts are improving safety and making a demonstrable difference. These and similar initiatives have not only improved outcomes and processes but also reduced reliance on fallible human functions while increasing the accessibility of consistent information. These are worthy efforts that should be sustained by all means. Yet they are only a portion of what can be done. The effort to increase patient safety by improving relationships between disciplines, departments, and patients is still noticeably absent as a strategy for improved safety. Without detracting from the recognition institutions have achieved for their improvements, it is also important to understand that the majority of that reform has focused on improving discipline-specific activities and functions carried out within defined boundaries. Few of the interventions have been directed to the improvement of cross-boundary processes or relationships.

Yet both intuitively and experientially, those of us in health care know that a large number of medical mishaps occur at boundary intersections. We also know that the quality of the relationships among the individuals involved in care plays a major role in determining the quality of care provided.

External Pressures for Reform and the Use of TQM

Concomitantly, external pressures continue to present a clear business case for an overall cultural transformation within health care institutions. Yet few safety initiatives except those related to error reporting are focusing on cultural change. Diminishing revenues and deficit bottom lines are stimulating health care organizations to transform themselves in multiple ways. Rebounding from the effects of times gone by, health care institutions must respond to an increasingly competitive environment and the demands of consumer and employer groups who are seeking better value. Many organizations have found that their leadership styles and employee behavioral characteristics will no longer sustain or move them to success.

The 1990s brought the revelation that many of the factors that made companies strong in the past would not keep them strong in the future (Levering & Moskowitz, 1993). Most pressing was the need to initiate a renewed sense of organizational membership among clinicians and nonclinicians. Inspiring organizational members to a higher calling was believed to be important to establishing a culture that would aid institutional success. The rapidity with which information was becoming available and regulatory and reimbursement requirements were changing heightened the necessity of orchestrating an organizational strategy for improvement. In addition, the emerging competition over quality of care provided a compelling impetus for change in the health care arena (Buerhaus, 1999).

Although institutions have used a variety of organizational and management strategies in response to evolving health care requirements, Total Quality Management (TQM) along with mission and values statements have been among the approaches most frequently embraced (Micklethwait & Wooldridge, 1996; Rigby, 1998). Collaboration, teamwork, and a more egalitarian spirit among organizational members are some important components of the TQM methodology. In the day-to-day care process and problem resolution, these concepts and principles are expected to reinforce a sense of collegiality and responsibility.

The TQM conceptual framework encourages institutions to value the voices and participation of all members. This model of shared leadership is an excellent first-line filter against clinical mishaps—that is, if it were fully embraced and put into practice. TQM concepts are widely accepted as theory; however, actual practice is following at a much slower pace. Several organizational factors impede the full actualization of this behavior.

Barriers to Reform

Anecdotal and documented information about individual and organizational barriers to improved error prevention are legendary (Leape, 1994; Arnold, 1998; Schulmeister, 1999). Among these barriers are the coveted sense of clinical autonomy among physicians, fear of malpractice litigation and punishment, inadequate dissemination and implementation of known safety practices and practice guidelines, and institutional hierarchies.

Clinical Autonomy

The concept of *clinical autonomy*, which is exercised by physicians in the treatment of their patients, is similar to the concept of academic freedom exercised by university faculty in the pursuit of pertinent knowledge and the teaching of that knowledge to their students. Clinical autonomy, like academic freedom, exists to allow professional and client needs to be met. In both cases, a service is provided, but at the same time undesired and unintended outcomes may occur. The inherent principles of both clinical autonomy and academic freedom enable and accommodate variability and thus also risk questionable practices. Clinical autonomy supports an environment of practice that is challenging to monitor or self-regulate.

Self-governance is an important component of the social contract between the medical profession and society in the United States. This contract grants authority over professional functions and permits autonomy in the conduct of the affairs of medicine. In return, the profession is expected to act responsibly, exercising self-regulation to ensure quality (American Nurses Association, 1980). Self-regulation, the core of the relationship between medicine and society, is an authentic hallmark of a mature profession. Medicine's standards of professional performance exist as established standards of practice, codes of ethics, and educational requirements for entry into professional practice. Although these standards have long served as a model for other groups working to achieve professional status, medicine's use of them to uphold its part of the social contract needs improvement.

The unwillingness of physicians to criticize each other's practices is a known and accepted behavior. Such reticence is understandable, particularly when viewed in the context of individuals who share responsibility for a professional domain and have economic linkages to each other. Rosenthal (1995) presents a comprehensive account of professional autonomy from the perspective of research subjects who are physicians and health care leaders. These physicians believe that clinical autonomy is necessary because a large part of medical work is "uncertain," driven by the interplay of patient care variables, organizational issues, and personal problems. Therefore, exercising independent judgment in care processes and strategy is not just a desirable professional attribute; it is believed to be necessary to good outcomes. The interviewees further acknowledged understanding their own fallibility and that of their colleagues. Because of their shared professional domain, they found it easy to identify with each other's actual experiences. This sense of shared vulnerability made it difficult for them to evaluate each other's practice behaviors critically. Such closely held beliefs also blur the boundaries between errors that are avoidable and those that are unavoidable, thus further confounding the willingness of physicians to share critical feedback or identify preventive strategies related to practice.

Fear of Malpractice Litigation

The threat of medical malpractice litigation is one of the most obvious barriers to the improvement of patient safety. The fact that action can be initiated for all kinds of errors, no matter how minor, has not only instilled a grave sense of fear in clinicians but has changed clinical practice and increased the cost of health care. Further, disclosing one's own error or a colleague's error poses the risk of financial ruin and loss of professional credibility. These risks also serve as disincentives to participate in improvement strategies to reduce the risk of error.

Fear of malpractice litigation and regulatory sanctions has also changed the relationships between patients and providers and resulted in new organizational pressures and changes (Gaucher & Coffey, 1993; Orlikoff & Vanagunas, 1988). This fear has undermined relationships by eroding trust and prompting defensive behaviors that result in needless expenses and unnecessary hospital administrative practices.

Inadequate Dissemination and Implementation of Safety Practices and Practice Guidelines

Known safety practices could significantly reduce the likelihood of error, yet many such practices remain unused. Why are these practices not implemented? What forces allow an organization or an individual to know yet resist or refrain from taking proven corrective action? The full answers to these questions are undoubtedly complex, involving both cultural and economic issues. However, because we know that health care individuals and organizations want to be the best and to do their best, it is obvious that this behavior is not due to a lack of caring.

Consider the institutional causes of adverse drug events, which make up a substantial portion of the total number of medical mishaps that occur during hospitalization (Bates et al., 1997). In a study by Leape et al. (1995) to identify and evaluate system factors that caused adverse drug events, drug dosing errors were found to occur significantly more often than other medication errors. The largest numbers occurred in the medication ordering stage, largely because orders were handwritten, illegible, and incomplete. These findings document issues that are as much a problem today as they were at the time of the study. Illegible and incomplete medication orders not only increase the cost of medication administration because of the extra time needed by pharmacists, clerks, and nurses to decipher the physician's intention; they also increase the risk of error and patient harm. Several elements contribute to this illegibility. Most orders are written in cursive rather than printed letters. Spelling may be inaccurate. Orders may employ personal abbreviations, symbols, and numbers. To avoid disruption of their workflow, nurses and pharmacists must try to learn the individual ordering idiosyncrasies of various physicians. The necessary and increasing use of supplemental personnel by hospital departments, particularly the nursing, clerical, and pharmacy services, compounds the inherent risks in these order-writing habits, creating further fertile ground for error. In addition to the illegibility of the order itself, another serious problem is illegible physician signatures. The nurse or pharmacist may not even be able to determine whom to call with a question regarding an order.

When a question does arise from illegibility, having to ask the question disrupts the questioner's flow of work and sometimes subjects that person to disrespectful responses from the prescriber, whose reaction is often an expression of frustration at having his or her own workflow interrupted for what he or she may consider an inconsequential question.

Individuals involved in processing and administering physician orders will follow those orders even when they do not comply with established policies because in general the policies do not specify the actions to be taken when an order does not comply. The processors also know that in practice, following policies is usually discretionary, whereas to fail to process the order means risking the wrath of both the physician who wrote the order and the nurse waiting to administer the order.

Aggressive responses from some prescribers intimidate nurses and pharmacists and encourage them to avoid clarifying questionable orders. Such responses gain immense institutional notoriety and thus can intimidate even those who have no direct interaction with these prescribers. Worse yet, this prescriber behavior, along with the tendency of nurses and pharmacists to accommodate such practices, unintentionally sends the message to any questioner that she or he is not as competent as colleagues who do not question. In reality, questioners raise the level of competency of all involved. However, the weight of the prevalent behavior within a culture is often very heavy and hard to resist. Before long the questioner becomes an expert accommodator, anticipating and acceding to the idiosyncrasies of the prescribers. Such accommodation further supports the culture of risk related to medical mishaps. In this climate, implementation of known, noncomplex safety practices is especially important.

The use of practice guidelines offers another avenue for safety, yet their use in many institutions also continues to be variable and discretionary. In the National Coalition on Health Care Report, Berwick (1998) makes the point that under- and overuse of therapies hinders practice and in the most egregious cases may cause harm. Examples of this problem include the variable use of beta blockers and aspirin to reduce the likelihood of death from heart attacks, inadequate use of steroid medications for asthma, the failure by primary care physicians to diagnose and treat depression, and the excessive use of antibiotics. In addition to encouraging medical mishaps, over- and underuse of therapies adds a tremendous expense to an already economically burdened system. Such practices continue at the same time as health care organizations are laying workers off to reduce expenses. Standardization is not a methodology that practitioners readily embrace, and their reasons for resisting deserve dialogue and intervention. Nevertheless, the lack of consistent practice encourages misuse and errors, and sometimes causes harm.

Hierarchical Relationships

The hierarchy of relationships in the hospital setting is one of the most profound barriers to safety practices. In no other relationship is this more observable than in the relationship of the nurse to the physician. Although the medical profession and the nursing profession each have their own patient care domains, a subset of the nursing response is driven by physician orders and treatment regimens. In spite of the fact that most nursing care can be provided independent of a physician's order and that nurses are legally and professionally accountable for the care they provide, many physicians believe that the doctor is completely and unquestionably responsible for all care provided. This belief, coupled with the administrative strategy of appointing physicians to administrative leadership roles in an effort to increase their institutional commitment and sense of shared ownership, has motivated some physicians to advocate for clinical and administrative authority over all care providers, including nurses. The typical institutional deference afforded physicians and the reputation for power and dominance associated with the practice of medicine support their demands for an authoritative role, one that is based on power and dominance rather than collaboration and a sense of teamwork. This institutional power structure promotes an environment of passivity and silence from nurses.

There is increasing evidence that nurse-physician collaboration is associated with improved patient outcomes (Doering, 1999; Fagin, 1992; Corley, 1998; Sovie, 1993; Lawry, 1995; Baggs et al., 1999; Edmondson, 1996). In spite of this evidence and the fact that institutions articulate a desire for empowered workers to cooperate in interdependent, complementary relationships, many nurses and doctors continue to carry out their roles in ways that support the traditional hierarchical relationships. In addition, the structure and the culture of most institutions support this tradition, the impact of which is apparent in striking ways.

Nurses have articulated and acted out a strong sense of hesitancy in challenging or questioning physician orders and practices. The increased attention to analyses of the root cause of medical mishaps has exposed the concern and intimidation that the staff nurse experiences when faced with questionable medical practices or orders. Corley (1998), in examining nurse-physician relationships in the critical care area, speaks to the impact of gender and prestige on nurse-physician relationships. Although the hand-maiden image of nurses has changed and the number of female physicians is increasing, the high percentage of female nurses and the high prestige of physicians affect the nature and quality of their communication. Corley documents nurses' perception that physicians do not value their opinions, as well as their fear of challenging a physician. This perception is one of the principal reasons that nurses prefer not to participate with physicians during patient care rounds. Many nurses say that because their input is rarely acknowledged by physicians or addressed in plans of care, making rounds is not an effective use of their time.

The sense of fear and intimidation is not without cause. Fagin (1992) explains eloquently the issues involved. The nursing and medical professions share a unique kinship that engenders a closeness that tends to blur differences in structure and priorities. In addition their domains of practice appear so related that they are often indistinguishable. These two factors reinforce a lack of visibility for nursing, even though the historical and legal basis of nursing is quite distinct from that of medicine. Often when conflict in relation to clinical practice arises over who controls what, the physician is considered the authority. The fact that nurses are considered employees and physicians entrepreneurs, responsible for the institutional revenue stream, tends to strengthen the physician's sense of ownership, diminishing the possibilities for the development of collegiality.

Finding themselves in physician-dominated hierarchies when care goes awry or their level of dissatisfaction escalates, nurses will exert considerable covert ingenuity to protect patients or express their displeasure. Indirect methods of expression are sought over more directly assertive methods because of the fear of being seen as disloyal. This indirect behavior is reinforced by the views of administrators that open expression of such dissatisfaction is disloyal and disruptive. So nurses learn to maintain a code of silence. This silence undermines interdisciplinary collegiality and interferes with a potential first-line filter for medical mishaps.

The Need for Cultural Transformation

In the day-to-day reality of the hospital environment, certain cultural factors reinforce and expand the risks related to adverse events. To change these conditions a profound cultural transformation is required. This cultural shift has to begin at the top of the organization and must have a positive effect on the behaviors of all organizational members. Culture is intrinsic to every organization. Simply stated, culture is the way things are done in a particular environment. The shared belief systems of the individuals within an organization form the ideological underpinnings of the culture (Zammuto, Gifford, & Goodman, 1999). The culture both shapes and is shaped by the behavior of the individuals within it. It is a broad force manifesting itself in all aspects of behavior, including the manner in which individuals communicate, interact, and work together. Culture defines a workgroup's priorities, power structure, and peer relationships and its willingness to change or resist change (Simms & Coeling, 1993).

Simms and Coeling (1993) liken culture to snow, in that, like a fall of snowflakes, culture covers everything. As each individual snowflake subtly settles into place, the effects of the cumulative snowstorm can be very powerful. The same holds true for culture. Each actual behavior may be subtle, yet the total effect of a group's culture is a powerful force. Therefore, all desired changes or innovations involving most behaviors are cultural changes; as such, they require more than a management pronouncement that change must occur. A carefully designed, integrated organizational strategy must be implemented, and it must recognize that everything is connected to everything.

Conclusion

A nonpunitive approach is an absolute requirement if a health care institution is to respond to errors in a manner that reinforces the successful implementation of improvement strategies, with the ultimate goal of safeguarding society. A culture of improvement that promotes disclosure and analysis of errors and near misses is critical to initiate the level of change needed. Creating an environment of trust and improvement does not mean that individual accountability has no place in the process. Accountability remains, and in those medical mishaps in which the cause is assessed to be reckless noncompliance with regulatory standards or laws, sanctions should follow.

Changing systems so they support appropriate behaviors through the use of policies and directives will decrease medical mishaps and increase patient safety. It will also inform and prepare the environment for the more fundamental, critical relationship changes that must be employed to ensure long-term safety.

References

American Nurses Association. (1980). *Nursing: A social policy statement*. Kansas City, MO: Author.

Arnold, G. J. (1998). Clinical recognition of adverse drug reactions: Obstacles and opportunities for the nursing profession. *Journal of Nursing Care Quality, 13*(2), 45–55.

Baggs, J. G., Schmitt, M. H., Mushlin, A. I., Mitchell, P. H., Eldredge, D. H., Oakes, D., & Hutson, A. D. (1999). Association between nurse-physician collaboration and patient outcomes in three intensive care units. *Critical Care Medicine, 27*(9), 1991–1998.

Banister, G., Butt, L., & Hackel, R. (1996). How nurses perceive medication errors. *Nursing Management, 27*(1), 31–34.

Bates, D. W., Spell, N., Cullen, D. J., Burdick, E., Laird, N., Petersen, L. A., Small, S. D., Sweitzer, B. J., & Leape, L. L. (1997). The costs of adverse drug events in hospitalized patients. *Journal of the American Medical Association, 277*, 307–311.

Berwick, D. (1998) *As good as it should get: Making healthcare better in the new millennium* (National Coalition on Health Care Report). Washington, DC: National Coalition on Health Care.

Buerhaus, P. (1999, April). *Trouble in the nurse labor market? Recent trends, outlook for future employment and earning, and prospects for a severe and sustained RN shortage*. Paper presented at the meeting of the University Health System Consortium, Chicago.

Corley, M. C. (1998). Ethical dimensions of nurse-physician relations in critical care. *Nursing Clinics of North America, 33*(2), 325–337.

Doering, L. V. (1999). Nurse-physician collaboration: At the crossroads of danger and opportunity. *Critical Care Medicine, 27*(9), 2066–2067.

Edmondson, A. C. (1996). Learning from mistakes is easier said than done: Group and organizational influences on the detection and correction of human error. *Journal of Applied Behavioral Science, 32*(1), 5–28.

Fagin, C. M. (1992). Collaboration between nurses and physicians: No longer a choice. *Academic Medicine, 67*(5), 295–303.

Gaucher, E. J., & Coffey, R. J. (1993). *Total quality in health care.* San Francisco: Jossey-Bass.

Grant, S. M. (1999). Who's to blame for tragic error? *American Journal of Nursing, 99*(9), 9.

Joint Commission on Accreditation of Healthcare Organizations (JCAHO). (1998). *Sentinel events: Evaluating cause and planning improvement* (2nd ed.). Oakbrook Terrace, IL: Author.

Kohn, L. T., Corrigan, J. M., & Donaldson, M. S. (Eds.); Committee on Quality of Health Care in America, Institute of Medicine. (2000). *To err is human: Building a safer health system.* Washington, DC: National Academy Press.

Lawry, T. C. (1995). Making culture a forethought: What to do when strategy meets organizational culture. *Health Progress, 76*(4), 22–25

Leape, L. L. (1994). Error in medicine. *Journal of the American Medical Association, 272,* 1851–1857.

Leape, L. L. (2000). Can we make healthcare safe? In S. Findlay (Ed.), *Reducing medical errors and improving patient safety: Success stories from the front lines of medicine* (pp. 2–3, A.C.T. for America's Health publication). Washington, DC: National Coalition on Health Care.

Leape, L. L., Bates, D. W., Cullen, D. J., Cooper, J., Demonaco, H. J., Gallivan, T., Hallisey, R., Ives, J., Laird, N., Laffel, G., Nemeskal, R., Petersen, L. A., Porter, K., Servi, D., Shea, B. F., Small, S. D., Sweitzer, B. J., Thompson, B. T., & Vander Vliet, M. (1995). Systems analysis of adverse drug events. *Journal of the American Medical Association, 274,* 35–43.

Levering, R., & Moskowitz, M. (1993). The one hundred best companies to work for in America. New York: Doubleday.

Micklethwait, J., & Wooldridge, A. (1996, September 30). The witch doctors. *New York Times.*

Moore, P. (1999). *A cultural assessment of a university health system operating room.* Consultant report, Ann Arbor, MI.

Orlikoff, J. E., & Vanagunas, A. (1988). *Malpractice prevention and liability control for hospitals* (2nd ed.). Chicago: American Hospital Publishing.

Paul, C. (2000). Back from the brink. In S. Findlay (Ed.), *Reducing medical errors and improving patient safety: Success stories from the front lines of medicine* (pp. 4–8, A.C.T. for America's Health publication). Washington, DC: National Coalition on Health Care.

Rebillot, K. (2000). Tackling medication errors head on. In S. Findlay (Ed.), *Reducing medical errors and improving patient safety: Success stories from the front lines of medicine* (pp. 18–20, A.C.T. for America's Health publication). Washington, DC: National Coalition on Health Care.

Reese, S. (2000) Making mistakes harder to make. In S. Findlay (Ed.), *Reducing medical errors and improving patient safety: Success stories from the front lines of medicine* (pp. 21–23, A.C.T. for America's Health publication). Washington, DC: National Coalition on Health Care.

Rigby, D. K. (1998, September 7). What's today's special at the Consultants Cafe? *Fortune*, pp. 162–163.

Rosenthal, M. M. (1995). *The incompetent doctor: Behind closed doors*. Bristol, PA: Open University Press.

Schulmeister, L. (1999). Chemotherapy medication errors: Descriptions, severity, and contributing factors. *Oncology Nursing Forum, 26*(6), 1033–1042.

Simms, M. L., & Coeling, V. E. (1993). Facilitating innovation at the nursing unit level through cultural assessment: How to keep management ideas from falling on deaf ears. *Journal of Nursing Administration, 23*(4), 46–53.

Smetzer, J. (1998). Beyond blaming individuals. *Nursing 98*, 48–51.

Sovie, M. D. (1993). Hospital culture: Why create one? *Nursing Economics, 11*(2), 69–75, 90.

Zammuto R. F., Gifford, B., & Goodman, E. A. (1999). *Managerial ideologies, organizational culture and the outcomes of innovation: A competing values perspective*. Manuscript submitted for publication.

5

The Patient's View of Medical Errors

Michael L. Millenson

Medical errors look different from the patient's side of the bed:

> The nurse came in and [because I'm a health care consultant] I asked, "Did they give my father his meds today?" It wasn't on the chart. It turns out they didn't give it to him.

> My mother had significantly elevated high blood pressure when she was initially admitted. Unfortunately, she was given the wrong medication. The medical care was clearly inadequate during her first few days. There is absolutely no question in my mind that my mother would not be alive today if I were not a physician and watching over every step of the care.

> As a physician, I know the chances of suffering a stroke during [a certain diagnostic procedure] are about one in 10,000. It turned out three women had suffered strokes in one week. After my wife [recuperated and] complained, the chief of radiology blamed the strokes on three women patients who were "nervous."

As part of the Hippocratic oath, every newly minted physician swears to uphold the fundamental principle, "First, do no harm." That, in a nutshell, is the patient's view of the entire medical errors debate: treat me, but treat me safely. Unfortunately, the culture of actual medical practice provides physicians with a far more ambivalent message. As medical sociologist Eliot Freidson (1970) wrote: "The benefit of the doubt is given to colleague performance. . . . 'After all,' the argument goes, 'nobody *wants* to kill a patient.' But if one does kill a patient, perhaps good intentions are not enough. So long as [the profession] emphasizes good intentions rather than good performance . . . the profession cannot really regulate itself" (p. 366).

This emphasis on good intentions rather than good performance may well be the most telling difference between the ways physicians and patients look at medical mistakes. Indeed, almost any sort of treatment decision has at one time or another been blithely justified under the *good intentions* rubric.

The Days of Good Intentions

In *The Silent World of Doctor and Patient*, Jay Katz (1984), himself a physician, related how it took a decision by the U.S. Supreme Court to guarantee a patient's simple right to know in advance what surgical procedure the doctor was planning to perform. The case involved a female patient with epilepsy who sued her surgeon for removing her uterus and ovaries without telling her his intentions in advance. The surgeon countered by saying he had deceived the patient so that she would not resist having a needed procedure. The Supreme Court sided with the patient, ruling in a 1905 opinion that even the most "eminent" physician or surgeon cannot violate a patient's body without prior consent. Nonetheless, it was not until the early 1970s that courts forced doctors to disclose not only the procedure to be performed, but also, in layperson's language, its likely benefits and possible harmful effects.

Along with emphasizing good intentions, physicians are prone to see a substantial chunk of medical mistakes as impervious to preventive action. As a prominent forensic medicine specialist put this argument back in the 1950s, 50 to 80 percent of malpractice suits could be eliminated if physicians would just stop criticizing each other's "unavoidable" errors (Regan, 1954). Similarly, a pathbreaking article on medical errors that also appeared in the 1950s concluded sadly that errors were the price to be paid for "the inestimable benefits of modern diagnosis and therapy" (Barr, 1955).

Yet even clearly preventable errors were not enough to prompt collegial correction. When sociologist Freidson (1970) asked doctors what they would do about a colleague whose behavior violated technical norms of conduct, the most common response was "nothing." Asked what they would do if the offense were repeated, doctors answered: "I'd talk to him." The various informal disciplinary techniques, concluded Freidson, "were never so strong as to reduce income and minimize or prevent work on the part of offenders, and they were rarely organized" (pp. 149, 151).

Hospital administrators have evinced similar circle-the-wagons behavior over the years. In 1943, a nationwide epidemic of diarrhea among newborns killed as many as two-thirds of the affected babies. However, hospital administrators did not seek assistance from local health departments in addressing the infection outbreaks because, as an investigator discovered, they feared bad publicity (Lembcke, 1943). This attitude of "see no evil" persisted into the 1970s, as physician gadfly Robert Mendelsohn (1979) related in a medical exposé of the period: "If you're in the operating room and somebody finds a sponge in the belly left from a previous operation, traditional ethics would make sure that somebody in the family found out about it. Medical ethics tells you to keep your mouth shut about it. The surgeon will say, 'I don't want anybody to know about this,' and if the nurse tells the family, she'll be out of a job" (p. 46).

Patients in the 1950s, often grateful just to have access to modern medical treatment, could be as forgiving toward doctors and hospitals as they were toward themselves. Still, there were no illusions about professional peccadilloes. As a *Fortune* article of that era put it: "The physician, after all, is organized into a guild whose rules require mutual back scratching and forbid face clawing. [But] so long as they do not violate guild rules and name names, they will even talk about the occasional incompetence and rascality in their profession" (Maurer, 1954, p. 179).

Public Views Change, Old Practices Persist

Indeed, medical mistakes began to emerge into public view due at least as much to societal changes as to professional ones. The social upheaval of the 1960s and 1970s emboldened dissident doctors to break the code of silence that provided "maximum autonomy for the individual physician . . . and little criticism from peers" (Stevens, 1989, p. 246). At the same time, patients started to lose their patience. Ralph Nader, who had gained fame by attacking the safety record of General Motors, formed the Public Citizen Health Research Group. The group's first (and current) executive director, Sidney Wolfe, M.D., soon became a favorite source for medical reporters. The group's stories helped, and are still helping, to fuel the public's demand for change.

Like the news media, the courts were also becoming less quiescent. Nonprofit hospitals had been immune to malpractice suits both because they were "charities" and because they presented themselves as essentially the doctor's workshop. The care of an eighteen-year-old Illinois boy who broke his leg in a football game changed that equation forever. Because of poor care by a doctor who had not set a fracture in three years, the boy's leg became infected and eventually had to be amputated. The hospital argued that it only provided a setting within which physicians practiced. The Illinois Supreme Court, however, ruled that patients who avail themselves of "hospital facilities" expect that the hospital will attempt to cure

them, not that the nurses and others "will act on their own responsibility" (*Darling* v. *Charleston Hospital*, 1965).

Not surprisingly, the growth of critical forces inside and outside
health care led to more, and more successful, malpractice suits. The
surge in judgments for the patients led to a debate over whether
this situation was due to poor doctoring or good lawyering. A physi-
cian-attorney named Don Harper Mills undertook a research effort
of unprecedented scope to answer that question. He sampled
20,864 medical charts, obtained from twenty-three California hospitals, in a search for "potentially compensable events"—a lawyerly
term for treatment-caused injuries. Mills (1978) concluded that
one patient in twenty was harmed by treatment. About four in
every hundred of these "events" caused major, permanent disability, and almost ten in every hundred resulted in the patient's death.
Although the percentages were small, they meant that California
hospital patients in 1974 suffered 140,000 treatment-caused injuries, including 13,600 hospital-caused fatalities.

The divergence of the patient and professional viewpoints is
clear in what happened next. The profession did not immediately
launch an all-out effort to reduce mistakes. Instead, Mills focused
on how well-intentioned practitioners were being victimized by patients who did not understand that errors were unavoidable. Mills
(1978) wrote: "*No one* should remain unaware that benefits and adverse risks [of modern medicine] are inseparable" (p. 365).

In any event, Mills's primary interest was in "potentially compensable events." Here, there was good news for doctors: even when
a patient suffered permanent disability or death, there was less than
a fifty-fifty chance of a successful lawsuit (Mills, 1978).

The 1970s surge of consumer activism led to some significant
changes. For example, the Joint Commission on Accreditation of
Healthcare Organizations completely overhauled its standards. Yet
in other ways the outrage of the era left a legacy no more durable
than a sand castle built at low tide. Consider: in 1974, an estimate

that as many as 30,000 to 140,000 hospital patients suffered fatal drug reactions every year became big news (Talley & Laventurier, 1974). Twenty-five years later, a similar estimate — 44,000 to 98,000 Americans killed each year by in-hospital errors — also became front-page news. This despite the admitted fact that much of the research for that estimate, contained in a report released in 1999 by the Institute of Medicine (Kohn, Corrigan, & Donaldson, 2000), came from a 1991 study that examined incidents that had occurred in 1984. That study had found a level of deaths very similar to the number reported by Mills in the 1970s (Brennan et al., 1991).

Absent consumer activism, the simple airing of somber facts has accomplished little. When the death of Libby Zion, the daughter of *New York Times* reporter Sidney Zion, was linked to treatment by tired, overworked medical residents, public outrage brought new laws limiting the number of hours worked by medical residents (albeit laws where both the compliance and the enforcement have been spotty). However, even though the 1986 grand jury report on the death called for major New York teaching hospitals to install computerized systems to prevent drug errors, that part of the report got no public attention and no provider action.

In late 1999, in the wake of the Institute of Medicine report on medical errors, a coalition of employers called the Leapfrog Group received front-page play in the *New York Times* for demanding that all hospitals install computerized drug-drug interaction systems. Neither journalists nor the employers, however, recalled the missed opportunities — the washed away sand castles — of the past.

It is tempting to regard malpractice suits as the ultimate patient answer to medical mistakes. In many respects this would be unfortunate. There is, after all, a genuine difference between doctors who are drunks, drug addicts, or mentally disturbed (delicately referred to by the profession as *impaired physicians*) or incompetent (*bad doctors*) and the 90 to 95 percent of doctors who are well trained and hard working and who sometimes make a mistake due to either human imperfection or badly designed systems. There is also a difference between a good decision poorly executed (accidentally giving a harmful dose of a beneficial drug) and a bad decision (prescribing a harmful drug).

Indeed, most malpractice suits could be avoided by timely disclosure of what went wrong and an apology. By some estimates, as many as 80 percent of malpractice cases are filed because of a breakdown in the patient-doctor relationship (Wu, 1999). One cannot help but wonder whether this is due to the belief by too many physicians that their failings are "unavoidable," and the patient's "expectations" are the real difficulty.

In any event, the malpractice system is as unlikely to redress most patient wrongs today as it was when Mills examined it a quarter century ago. A 1997 study in a Chicago teaching hospital, for example, found that 18 percent of patients suffered a serious adverse event related to their care, yet only 1 percent of patients filed a claim for compensation (Andrews et al., 1997). Yet in many ways, the lawsuit has been the only lever patients have possessed. Although the malpractice system is roundly detested and feared by doctors, a historian of U.S. malpractice litigation notes that "from the public's point of view . . . halting efforts to guarantee standards among various subsets of physicians themselves proved quickly and utterly ineffectual. . . . The only alternative for patients was to try to hold individual practitioners, one at a time, to whatever standards they or their lawyers, one at a time, wanted to impose" (Mohr, 2000). From the patient's point of view, after all, the origin of a medical mistake makes little difference. Indeed, hospitals and medical staffs have arguably paid more attention to impaired practitioners, where the legal risk is obvious, than to fixing systems errors that lack an easy villain.

To give just one example: by 1994, Salt Lake City's LDS Hospital was reporting that it had eliminated seven out of ten possible adverse drug events through a computerized monitoring system (R. Scott, personal communication, June 1995). (Some problems, like a previously undiagnosed patient drug allergy, cannot be anticipated.) To put that achievement into context, the 1991 Harvard Medical Practice Study—the study on which much of the IOM report was based—concluded that four out of ten errors in administering a drug could be prevented. In other words, LDS Hospital's record surpassed this supposed ideal (Millenson, 1997). Yet computerized drug monitoring is only now coming to the forefront, thanks to a combination of economic and public pressures and technological advances.

The Promise of Effective Change in Practices

Despite this grim history, there is room for optimism. The patient's perspective is being increasingly considered. Perhaps the defining event in this change was a page one article in the Sunday, March 23, 1995, issue of the *Boston Globe* (Knox, 1995). In heartbreaking detail the story related how Betsy Lehman, a young mother of two and a *Globe* medical columnist, had been painfully killed by an accidental drug overdose during treatment for breast cancer at Boston's renowned Dana-Farber Cancer Institute.

Just a few months before the *Globe* article appeared—and before a spate of other headline-grabbing mistakes—medical errors were nowhere to be found on either the policy or professional agenda. Indeed, an article and accompanying commentary in the *Journal of the American Medical Association* bemoaned the profession's "ostrichlike" attitude. As the commentator put it: "Mistakes have been treated as uncommon and atypical, requiring no remedy beyond the traditional . . . [even though] a large and growing collection of literature demonstrates that physicians' approaches to the management of medical error do not work well enough (Blumenthal, 1994, p. 1867).

The Lehman incident, however, made it unavoidably clear that even the best-trained doctors desperately needed information systems help. At Dana-Farber, a premier cancer hospital, a computerized order-entry system would have stopped the doctor who mistakenly thought that the dose of the anticancer drug cisplatin meant to be given over a four-day period was to be given *each* day for four days.

In Massachusetts, hospitals and others reacted to the Lehman tragedy by forming the Coalition for the Prevention of Medical Errors. Separately, the Joint Commission on Accreditation of Healthcare Organizations has introduced new rules for reporting errors that encourage hospitals to make improvements based on *root cause analysis* of mistakes. The American Hospital Association and the American Medical Association (AMA) have begun talking openly about medical mistakes, working with the nonprofit Institute for Healthcare Improvement.

Within a year of the Lehman incident, the AMA had radically changed its public pronouncements about medical mistakes and had helped set up the National Patient Safety Foundation. The foundation is charged with funding research into error prevention and disseminating information on ways to prevent errors. In addition, the foundation's founding executive director left to form another group with similar goals, the National Partnership for Patient Safety.

Just as important is the way the Lehman case raised the profile of medical errors in the news media. Even before the December 1999 IOM report, the news media were paying closer attention to the debate over the causes of medical mistakes, in publications ranging from *USA Today* (Davis, 1998) to *The New Yorker* (Gawande, 1999) to *Worth* magazine, where a freelance journalist wrote an agonizing account of the death of his wife and newborn son due to poor care by a well-known obstetrician at a respected New York hospital (Grossman, 1997–1998).

After Lehman's death, the news media, regulators, and legislators also interacted to enhance patient power. For example, the availability of state-collected information on errors in Massachusetts gave *Boston Globe* reporter Larry Tye ammunition for a follow-up series on medical errors that highlighted ongoing problems. Similarly, regulatory requirements connected with the sale of a major Pennsylvania hospital jump-started the award-winning 1999 series on medical errors written by the *Philadelphia Inquirer's* Andrea Gerlin. The print media, in turn, provided some examples of "real human beings" that were used in the IOM report and by broadcast media and politicians reacting to that report.

At the same time, consumer groups have been joined in their advocacy on this issue by real consumers. Karen Burton, an Iowa woman who had sued unsuccessfully to get a major teaching hospital to reveal its nosocomial infection rate, posted the results of her trials and tribulations on a Web site for others to learn from. Patricia Donnelly, a Queens, New York, woman who lost a young grandson to incompetent anesthesia administration during minor surgery, started a newsletter and one-woman lobbying campaign for greater disclosure of specific malpractice information. Indeed, the Internet, with its ability to shine a continuing light into previously hidden areas, may yet be the patient's greatest ally.

Major employers are also starting to become involved in this issue for the first time as they realize that the lives—and money— saved belong to their employees and their families. Gateway Purchasers for Health, in St. Louis, organized a seminar in May 2000 designed to call "urgent" attention to the "human and dollar cost of medical errors." DaimlerChrysler Corporation executives noted that the human cost of medical mistakes amounts to "one death of a DaimlerChrysler employee, dependent, or retiree every other day." Meanwhile, the magazine *Business & Health* bluntly titled an April 1, 2000, article on this topic: "Do American Hospitals Get Away with Murder?"

Legislators, always attuned to constituent concerns, have also become more vocal. IOM recommendations to establish the Center for Patient Safety within the Agency for Healthcare Research and Quality and to require mandatory error reporting quickly sparked congressional hearings. And because the public does not differentiate between a *systems error* and an *incompetent doctor* type of fatal mistake, there is also renewed interest in legislation to open to the public the confidential National Practitioner Data Bank, which documents significant disciplinary actions against doctors. Meanwhile, the Florida legislature and others state legislatures have held hearings highlighting the human face of medical mistakes.

There is room to hope that this time, doctors and hospitals will both listen and change. In Pittsburgh a group of prominent chief executive officers of major corporations succeeded in early 2000 in persuading local hospitals, doctors, and health plans to agree to an extraordinarily ambitious goal: eliminating all preventable drug errors and nosocomial infections. The CEOs were themselves lobbied by the Pittsburgh Regional Healthcare Initiative, a nonprofit organization with strong business leadership (Robinet, 2000).

Still, many doctors and hospitals continue to believe that this latest furor over errors is overblown. Reduce hospital-caused infections? Our people are well trained and hard working, a Minneapolis physician told me; perhaps the infection rate could be tweaked 1 or 2 percent lower. (The medical literature suggests a 50 percent reduction is achievable.) Computerized order-entry systems? Not a bad idea, the medical leadership of a Chicago hospital responded, but the hospital should be reimbursed for the expense. And anyway, what about the lawyers? As a commentator put it in the *New England Journal of Medicine* in a warning about making too much of the IOM report: "To address the problem of iatrogenic injuries seriously, we must reform the system of malpractice litigation" (Brennan, 2000, p. 1125).

Perhaps. Or perhaps, tragically, it will take even more litigation for the patient's voice to finally be heard loud and clear. As Ralph Nader might put it, the health care system is too often "unsafe at any speed."

Jack Risenhoover, general counsel of Eclipsys Corporation, a Delray Beach, Florida, company that sells computerized order-entry systems, sums up the choice this way:

The liability of *not* utilizing such technology is staggering and inevitable. Historically, it's similar to what happened in other industries that were slow to adopt
available technology to protect public health and safety.
    In a profession whose fundamental tenet is "First, do
no harm," reducing avoidable medical errors should be
priority one.[1]

That principle, rather than arguments about lawsuits, ought to
be the final word.

Note

1. See the Eclipsys Web site [www.eclipsnet.com/external/company/
   00%2D09webseminars.htm].

References

Andrews, L. B., Stocking, C., Krizek, T., Gottlieb, L., Krizek, C., Vargish, T.,
    & Siegler, M. (1997, February 1). An alternative strategy for studying ad-
    verse events in medical care. *Lancet, 349*, 309–313.
Barr, D. (1955). Hazards of modern diagnosis and therapy: The price we pay.
    Journal of the American Medical Association, 159, 1452–1456.
Blumenthal, D. (1994). Making medical errors into medical treasures. *Journal of
    the American Medical Association, 272*, 1867–1868.
Brennan, T. A. (2000). The Institute of Medicine report on medical errors:
    Could it do harm? *New England Journal of Medicine, 342*, 1123–1125.
Brennan, T. A., Leape, L. L., Laird, N. M., Herbert, L. E., Localio, A. R.,
    Lawthers, A. G., Newhouse, J. P., Weiler, P. C., & Hiatt, H. H. (1991).
    Incidence of adverse events and negligence in hospitalized patients:
    Results of the Harvard Medical Practice Study I. *New England Journal
    of Medicine, 324*, 370–376.
Darling v. Charleston Hospital, 33 Ill. 2d 326, 211 N.E. 2d 253 (1965).
Davis, R. (1998, October 19). Medicine's flying lessons: Aviation's safety pre-
    scriptions land in operating rooms. *USA Today*, p. D1.
Freidson, E. (1970). *The profession of medicine: A study of the sociology of applied
    knowledge*. New York: HarperCollins.
Gawande, A. (1999, February 1). When doctors make mistakes. *The New Yorker*,
    pp. 40–55.

Grossman, E. (1997, December–1998, January). The best medicine. *Worth*,
    pp. 98–122.

Katz, J. (1984). *The silent world of doctor and patient*. New York: Free Press.

Knox, R. A. (1995, March 23). Doctor's orders killed cancer patient. *Boston
    Globe*, p. 1-1.

Kohn, L. T., Corrigan, J. M., & Donaldson, M. S. (Eds.); Committee on Quality
    of Health Care in America, Institute of Medicine. (2000). *To err is human:
    Building a safer health system*. Washington, DC: National Academy Press.

Lembcke, P. A. (1943). Prevention and control of epidemic diarrhea is the ad-
    ministrator's responsibility. *Modern Hospital, 60,* 98–102.

Maurer, H. (1954, February). The MD's are off their pedestal. *Fortune*, pp. 139–
    142, 176, 179–180, 182, 184, 186.

Mendelsohn, R. S. (1979). *Confessions of a medical heretic*. Chicago:
    Contemporary.

Millenson, M. L. (1997). *Demanding medical excellence: Doctors and accountability
    in the information age*. Chicago: University of Chicago Press.

Mills, D. H. (1978, April). Medical Insurance Feasibility Study: A technical
    summary. *Western Journal of Medicine, 128,* 360–365.

Mohr, J. C. (2000). American medical malpractice litigation in historical per-
    spective. *Journal of the American Medical Association, 283,* 1731–1737.

Regan, L. J. (1954). Medicine and the law. *New England Journal of Medicine,
    250,* 463–467.

Robinet, J. E. (2000, April 14–20). Health initiative aims to balance competi-
    tion, community interests: Committee includes leaders of industry,
    health, and labor. *Pittsburgh Business Times*, p. 1.

Stevens, R. (1989). *In sickness and in wealth*. New York: Basic Books.

Talley, R. B., & Laventurier, M. F. (1974). Drug-induced illness. *Journal of the
    American Medical Association, 229,* 1043.

Wu, A. W. (1999). Handling hospital errors: Is disclosure the best defense? *An-
    nals of Internal Medicine, 131,* 970–972.

Part Three

Approaches to Managing Error

Concern with the quality of health care is not a new phenomenon. Substantial investments over the last few decades have been made to try to protect health care organizations and their members, through the development of clinical risk management programs, for example. At the same time, the medical knowledge base has experienced an enormous increase, with serious research efforts being targeted both toward understanding how the financing and delivery of health care might influence quality and toward developing more efficacious forms of treatment in the form of practice guidelines.

In Part Three, Chapters Six, Seven, and Eight provide a glimpse into these efforts, reviewing the claims and achievements of *error management*, *risk management*, *evidence-based medicine*, and *outcomes research*.

The vice president and chief medical officer for a managed care organization suggests that controlling variation through standard practices is an important mechanism for mitigating error and describes current ways of fostering these practices. A team of risk managers describes the revolution in the risk management function as its focus has shifted from minimizing costs to improving quality and protecting patients. And a team of researchers studying clinical practice improvement (CPI) proposes that this approach can lead to more effective and safe practices that can be broadly applied.

An additional compelling theme running through this section is that as important as standard approaches are for controlling variation and improving quality, there is also a challenge for health care professionals in understanding when standards fit and when they do not.

6

Error Management and Patient Safety
A Managed Care Competency

Derek van Amerongen

For years, managed care organizations (MCOs) have pursued as part of their fundamental value proposition the standardization of medical practice. From the beginning of the managed care movement in the early 1970s, it was clear that most physicians practiced in an independent, almost idiosyncratic manner (Phelps, 1992). The result has been a wide variation in approaches to clinical conditions. The same patient might get several significantly different recommendations from different physicians, and different patients with different diseases might get the same advice. In these circumstances, outcomes and quality management were necessarily problematic. The theory was that by bringing some sort of order to this confusion of treatments, the disease burden of a population would become more manageable and predictable.

This chapter describes the current approaches of MCOs toward establishing this order through standardization of practice and error management, offers a sampling of results, and suggests the issues still to be resolved.

The Current Status of Clinical Practice in the Community

We are now well into the second decade of managed care in the United States. It continues to evolve, as all processes should. Indeed, managed care in 2000 looks very different from the health maintenance organizations of the mid-1980s. Yet the picture of clinical practice in the community still reflects many of the elements that contribute to, if not foster, error in medicine. Despite the attempts of MCOs to educate physicians on the importance of reducing variations in practice, many clinicians continue to lack an appreciation of the role variations play in preventing better patient outcomes. These variations continue to exist in most clinical areas (Gross, Nicholson, & Powe, 1999), not only affecting care but also making it difficult for observers such as MCOs to accurately track processes across practice settings and medical groups. Certainly, unique patient characteristics will dictate customization of treatments when appropriate. However, when there is no medical rationale for differences in rates of surgeries, choices of medications, and the like, variation is neither desirable nor beneficial.

This situation is complicated by the lack of technological support in many medical providers' workplaces. Although personal computers and electronic communications have become routine for the average American, as of 1998, 59 percent of physicians did not have Internet access in their offices. This figure was actually an increase from 58 percent the year before. In 1999, 85 percent of hospitals submitted claims electronically to insurance companies and to the government; only 43 percent of physicians did so (McCormack, 2000). This discrepancy highlights more than the lack of business efficiency in the average medical practice. It is not just a question of how to generate bills but of how to keep current with new medical advances and how best to handle the huge volume of patient data. When they are not part of the explosion in electronic information sharing, physicians are unable to leverage the computer tools to improve their information management and better understand their practice. Given that the fundamental commodity in medicine is information, this failure has prevented the medical community from matching the kind of outcome improvements seen in other disciplines. It also creates an environment in which variation can persist, and with it, error.

Perhaps the element that most predisposes medical practitioners to perpetuate variation and hence increase the chance for error is the philosophy of medicine itself. Despite the changes in the health care landscape over the last decade, many physicians still seem to adhere to a cottage industry mentality. More than half of all physicians in the United States are in solo practice. Consequently, they have little opportunity for the kind of meaningful peer interaction that could change practice habits and address sources of error, even though evidence indicates that physicians work more safely and effectively in teams (Lawrence, 2000). Lack of appropriate interaction is also found among hospital-based clinicians and, indeed, is an issue in hospitals themselves. It is routine for physicians in academia, for example, to pass their entire careers in a single institution, from medical school through training and into practice. It is unheard of for a physician or hospital administrator to spend any significant time in other offices or hospitals just sitting, observing, and learning. Such behavior is a standard convention in industry, with cross-fertilization occurring between competitors and even between different industries, all with the goal of learning new techniques and avoiding stagnation. Medicine is perhaps the last industry in America to enshrine the silo as a business model. As a result, not only is the influence of technological innovations such as the Internet and electronic data management diluted but the far-reaching perspective essential to understanding what causes errors and how to deal proactively with them is absent.

The Managed Care Perspective

If the point of view of the provider is limited, what is that of the MCO? By necessity, the MCO sees the world in a larger context. Four key features are driving this shift away from the silo view of the physician, the medical practice group, and the hospital:

MCOs *are regional or national.* MCOs typically span a substantial geographical region. With the current mergers among the large

MCOs, one may speak of national (such as Humana) and regional plans (many Blue Cross plans), and even a combination of the two (such as groupings of regional plans). An MCO must have a broad base if it is to fulfill one of its primary functions, that of building a network of providers. This network needs to be diverse and offer access for the membership. It must also satisfy the demands of the corporate clients who contract with the MCO to provide benefits to their employees (van Amerongen, 1998). This means the MCO must have knowledge of the care patterns in a region and the providers. It must work with those providers to create insurance products that will deliver on its commitments to the payers. Once a network is designed and implemented, it must then be managed. This involves regular review of the adequacy of the network to meet member needs, collection of provider performance data, interactions with the providers to share the data and address problems, and so forth (Robinson, 1999). Consistency is vital. No employer wants to think that employees will receive significantly different care when they live in different areas. All providers expect, rightly, to be treated in the same manner and to have the same requirements apply to all. These necessary activities and approaches lead the MCO to view the various providers and covered populations from a much different standpoint than a physician takes when viewing a patient. Indeed, some of the conflict between MCOs and physicians revolves around these differing accountabilities: one is responsible for a population and one is responsible for an individual. Providers, even in the form of large medical groups and health systems, will never be able to match the MCO's population-wide scope, nor should they.

MCOs *are consumer oriented.* Managed care came into existence because employers and consumers of medical care recognized that the value proposition in U.S. medicine was fatally flawed: trillions of dollars were being spent without generating significant increases in health status (Anderson, 1997). Service was poor. Access was erratic. Satisfaction in general was low. In the 1992 presidential election, health care was a major topic, perhaps for the first time in any national election. Concern was focused mainly on the cost of care, although since then many other issues have emerged. Payers are now demanding numerous things from the system: broad networks with wide access, inclusion of most area hospitals, representation of all subspecialties, even alternative medicine coverage (Marber, 2000). These needs reflect the evolution of payers' expectations of health care. Meeting these needs is critical if there is to be any public support of health policy change. The question then becomes which component of the delivery system is most sensitive to the shifting desires of consumers, and which one can best drive the entire system in the direction consumers want. MCOs possess a broad perspective, as noted earlier. They are thus best situated to understand what the marketplace is asking for and how to respond. In the area of patient safety, seeing trends is particularly important, and trends are best appreciated at the MCO's broad level as opposed to the practitioner's level. An individual physician, nurse, or hospital may not realize the full significance of adverse events seen in isolation. A provider is also less concerned with the objectives of an employer who is obliged to satisfy a much larger constituency. For this reason, few medical practices have made the major modifications that would be necessary to place customer satisfaction at the center of their business model. Rather the patient is typically expected to adapt to the characteristics of the practice; if this is not acceptable, the patient usually finds another physician. Health plans must operate much differently to survive.

MCOs are technology based. Today it is impossible for a company of any size to do business without being part of the e-commerce world. The one exception to this rule is the medical practice (Bazzoli, 2000). It is a common experience to visit a group practice of five to seven physicians, generating several million dollars in revenue annually, and be unable to find a computer except for an older model used by the billing clerk. Without the aid of a computer, using such medical management tools as routine identification of high-risk patients or certain disease categories becomes exceedingly difficult. Of course a system that is largely nonautomated also increases the potential for error. Part of the isolation of the physician from the avalanche of new technology is due to insulation provided by the MCO itself as well as by the government and hospitals, who have made it possible for this one segment of the economy to function nonelectronically. Nevertheless, this isolation underscores the MCO's status as the entity best positioned to understand the complexity of systems and to have the tools to address that complexity.

MCOs *are market driven.* In this era of managed care bashing, this attribute may seem a negative one. Yet the necessity to be customer focused and to respond to the demands of the market forces the MCO to be an aggressive adopter of new technology and to deal rapidly with such customer concerns as patient safety. It also places the MCO in the role of facilitator between customer, member, and provider. MCOs have extensive experience in communicating with members and employers and with physicians. This is part of their basic function as required by the National Committee for Quality Assurance (NCQA, the accrediting agency for health plans) and by state and federal regulations. Skill in communication is essential for reducing error.

Imperatives Compelling MCOs to Address Error Aggressively

Systems design is a core competency of MCOs. Systems focus is key to ensuring patient safety. This concept is an old one in industry. W. Edwards Deming stated back in the 1950s that 85 percent of errors are attributable to systems and not to individuals (Duncan, 1995). If we accept his statement, which is the basis for such quality improvement programs as six sigma, then we must devote resources to this part of the problem, and focus on the areas that have the greatest opportunities for building error-reducing processes. Other industries have used systems analysis successfully to reduce error. For example, U.S. commercial aviation has seen fatalities decline from 1.18 per million departures in 1950 to 0.27 in 1990 (Lawrence, 2000). This result rests on analysis of data from multiple points of view to identify deviations from standard practices. These deviations are then studied to discover the system faults that permitted them to occur. This process is diametrically opposed to the traditional approach to quality assurance in medicine, in which a physician experiences an adverse event and is then dealt with in a punitive manner, with no attention given to learning whether the event represents an isolated episode that statistical probability tells us will occur periodically, or is part of a trend revealing a systems issue (such as poor technique, inadequate patient selection, problems with the operative equipment, and so forth). Thinking of such clinical situations as *systems issues* is a quantum change for most health care workers.

Leape (1994) identifies several aviation industry practices that could, with modification, prove useful in improving safety in medical settings:

- Aircraft designers assume that errors are inevitable and design systems to *absorb* them, building in buffers, automation, and redundancies.

- Procedures are standardized to the maximum extent possible, with specific protocols for operations, maintenance, and the like.

- The training and certification process is rigorous, highly developed, and frequently enforced.

- Safety is institutionalized, with oversight from two independent agencies (the Federal Aviation Administration and the National Transportation Safety Board). Recognizing that pilots seldom reported errors when such reporting led to disciplinary action, the FAA now has a confidential reporting system that has dramatically increased reporting. By placing accountability at an institutional level, the punitive aspects of error tracking and analysis are diminished, reporting is improved, and error reduction is effected.

In efforts of this kind, indicators used to evaluate systems must be measurable. They must also relate to meaningful outcomes. It is not beneficial to emphasize process measures that do not substantially reflect something about patient outcomes. MCOs have been involved in indicator development for the disease state management programs that are the hallmark of managed care plans (and required for NCQA accreditation). For instance, effectiveness in caring for obstetrical patients can be assessed in part by tracking the rates of HIV screening, prescription fills for prenatal vitamins, and so on. These intermediate process indicators serve as useful proxies for appropriate care.

Value creation is what payers seek when they contract with a health plan, just as they do when doing business with any supplier. Managed care is still building its track record on delivering value to its customers. Plans have been successful in establishing disease state management programs that seek to identify and work with patients with certain high-risk, chronic diseases. For example, according to the American Association of Health Plans *1999 Industry Survey*, almost 92 percent of managed health plans nationwide provide diabetic members with a trained diabetes care manager. Through a care management program, Humana was able to exceed the benchmarks for care for end-stage renal dialysis patients established by the U.S. Renal Data System. But as premiums began to rise again in 1999, employers were asking why they should pay more for the same products. Hence, if managed care can leverage its competency in managing systems to reduce error and return value to its customers, this will address a vexing question. It will also give consumers a reason to stick with health plans. Effective systems management also offers MCOs a chance to draw a clear distinction between managed care and the traditional medical delivery system based on an indemnity model.

Employers feel a definite sense of urgency about this issue. They know from experience that aggressive attention to systems problems leads to positive results, so it has become difficult for quality experts in industry to understand why medicine has been resistant to adopting appropriate systems management methods. General Motors, the largest payer for private medical care in the world, has publicly asked why proven solutions to medical errors — such as computerized drug dispensing systems — are not put into practice (Moore, 2000). There is frankly no acceptable reason why this has not been done. In other circumstances, such as air safety or food safety, it is difficult to imagine the public and government would tolerate thousands of deaths per year without immediate and radical action to prevent them. For GM, the 98,000 deaths per year attributed to medical error (Kohn, Corrigan, & Donaldson, 2000) translate into 9 GM beneficiaries dying each week. As large employers' patience with providers grows thin, so too does their patience with the health plans that presumably are actively managing the networks in which the providers practice.

MCOs would do well to adopt three targets for error reduction proposed by the Institute of Medicine report (Agency for Healthcare Policy and Research, 2000) and to add a fourth one:

1. Decrease error by 50 percent in five years.

2. Create systems to prevent recurrence.

3. Provide information to consumers.

4. Become a resource for providers.

One Health Plan's Approach

Anthem Blue Cross and Blue Shield is the largest Blue Cross plan in the nation. Through a series of mergers and acquisitions, it has become the largest health insurer in six of the eight states in which it owns the local Blues plan (Ohio, Indiana, Kentucky, New Hampshire, Connecticut, and Maine). Anthem Midwest serves the three states in which Anthem originally began. It is instructive to see the efforts Anthem has underway in that three-state region of Ohio, Indiana, and Kentucky, efforts that show how a plan can begin to manage error effectively and modify provider behavior to augment patient safety.

Anthem's philosophy in the Midwest has been to motivate and educate both providers and members to understand the issue of patient safety, and to improve systems to support that safety. This education occurs along several tracks. For members, education is carried out via newsletters, a Web site, and employer-based programs. This is nothing innovative, although it is an important function. The real opportunity comes through the Hospital Quality Program (HQP). An essential part of the HQP is an annual survey of every hospital that does managed care business with Anthem. Information is gathered from over three hundred hospitals across the three-state region. A request for information (RFI) is sent to each hospital prior to contracting for the coming year, asking the hospital to respond to several hundred indicators. A passing score is required before a managed care contract can be executed with the hospital. Thus the HQP has a unique ability to direct a hospital's attention to areas that are important to Anthem's quality efforts and to encourage the hospital to commit resources. The aggregate results of the RFI are shared with employers and members to help them understand global care patterns across the region. By requesting information at the hospital level, the emphasis on systems rather than individual practitioners is preserved. The hospital is motivated in turn to bring the medical staff into the quality improvement cycle to help correct deficiencies.

Anthem's research has mirrored that of other organizations in identifying significant sources of medical error. Knowing these sources suggests the kind of modifications that are most likely to work. According to the Agency for Healthcare Research and Quality (Bates et al., 1999), important sources of error in the delivery system are

- Inaccurate information recall, by both staff and patients.

- Diagnostic inaccuracies. These may arise from lack of familiarity with medical conditions (due to lack of experience), poor knowledge of proven therapies, and the like.

- Medication errors. The ordering and the administering of drugs are responsible for 56 percent and 34 percent of preventable adverse drug events, respectively. Dosage errors due to insufficient physician knowledge about the drug or the patient are also responsible for these errors.

With the documentation of these sources of error, the HQP goal is to design initiatives to address them.

Evaluating and Credentialing Participating Providers

Anthem focuses on providers in two target groups: hospitals and physicians. The hospital group is approached through the HQP review. The approach to physicians is directed in part through the HQP, insofar as the hospitals are expected to have a high level of medical staff input and commitment. However, the credentialing process for physicians involves a separate assessment of office capabilities and practice patterns (including a site review). Part of that review includes questions on patient safety measures. The goal is to make the two evaluations complementary and to convey a clear message about the need for physician involvement and attention to the safety issue.

The HQP surveys the following aspects of the hospital's proficiency in running error-minimizing systems. The key questions are designed both to inform Anthem of the hospital's progress in this area and to direct the institution toward quality improvement opportunities.

1. Use of electronic medicine:
   - Electronic medical record (EMR): how robust is the EMR? who has access? what is done to preserve patient confidentiality?
   - Exchange of data across different clinical areas: what is the level of ability to integrate patient data to prevent redundancies and avoid transmitting incorrect data?
   - Use of electronic order entry: what capabilities exist for implementing order entry in the EMR? what programs exist for implementing physician order entry to reduce error rates (see McDonald, 1999)? what, in detail, is the level of physician involvement and support of the process?
   - Use of standardized systems to report coded clinical information (in light of research highlighting inconsistent coding as an important cause of hospital misinformation and error, American College of Obstetricians and Gynecologists, 1994).
   - Integration of clinical guidelines into care patterns: how does the hospital translate guidelines from theory into bedside care?
   - Role of pharmacists in the intensive care unit: what is pharmacists' level of input during physician rounds in the ICU and in the acute care units? what is the level of review of medication orders by clinical pharmacists?
   - Role of the Patient Safety/Medical Errors Committee: does such a committee exist? how often does it meet? what is its purview in the hospital quality improvement

structure? what are the top five initiatives it undertook in the past year? In addition:

Discuss the strategic goals of the committee.

Describe the specific actions executed by the committee (for example, a review and analysis of all patient falls).

2. Tracking of medication errors: how is it done? how is the information used in the quality cycle? what, in detail, is the system that checks for dispensing errors in the pharmacy and again on the floor before the patient is dosed and that identifies gaps in prescription practice?

3. Process for encouraging reporting of errors by employees and physicians: what specific efforts are in place to remove the fear of reporting?

For physicians the following additional information is collected through the credentialing process. These data are then meshed with hospital data to create as complete a picture as possible of the clinical environment in a community:

1. Use of electronic data in the office setting.

2. Participation in hospital initiatives identified on the HQP.

3. Use of electronic claims submission to Anthem. (Although use of this tool is not a primary quality initiative, it is an important step in promoting office automation, helping physicians to overcome reluctance to use computer tools in their practice.)

Benchmarking: Sharing Data with Providers to Guide Systems Development

Medicine is often portrayed as a combination of art and science. The fact that deviation from guidelines and best practices results in thousands of deaths per year illustrates the need to make sure that the science side of this partnership is strong enough to reduce error in the day-to-day activities of most practitioners. Frequently the problem in applying scientific knowledge well is a lack of benchmarks to use with indicators. Anthem has sought to pair indicators with data that allow comparisons across groups and permit accurate profiling of hospitals and other providers. By identifying common reference points, drawn, ideally, from the scientific literature and endorsed by reputable third parties such as professional societies, outcomes can be both tracked and properly understood. Benchmarks serve multiple purposes:

- They increase the accountability of providers for outcomes.

- They permit providers to map their progress against a standard, ideally a quantitative one.

- They permit the MCO to identify outliers among providers at the earliest opportunity, so the plan can work with them in a proactive manner to improve results.

- They allow employers to compare plans and providers more easily, even when plan quality initiatives are different.

Commonality of data definitions is critical to defining care patterns, which in turn are needed to ensure patient safety. Before Anthem made the HQP information available to the medical community, virtually no hospital in the plan knew exactly how it measured up against its peers. Hospitals often did not know which parameters health plans were interested in, how these parameters were monitored, and how the hospitals could affect them and raise the level of quality care. Only a health plan, with its regional focus and a large pool of data, could deliver a uniform report, with all participants measured against a common standard. Once they have a better realization of the end effects of their processes, hospitals become better equipped to modify those processes to avoid errors and achieve optimal results.

Partnering with large employers is a valuable strategy in making this change occur. Employers are taking an increasingly active role in working with local health care providers as they see ever-larger portions of their revenue devoted to medical care, especially in communities where one or several employers loom large as payers. In Anderson, Indiana, for example, a city of 55,000 people, there are 18,000 GM and Delphi beneficiaries. Anderson, located thirty miles northeast of Indianapolis, had long experienced a hysterectomy rate that was the highest in the *world* for General Motors employees. GM undertook a unique partnership with the major health plans in the area, the two hospitals, and the physician groups, and benchmarking was done. High-volume physicians were identified and worked with to increase their adherence to the hysterectomy guidelines of the American College of Obstetricians and Gynecologists (Hallam, 2000). Patients were educated on common gynecological conditions and the range of options available, both surgical and nonsurgical. Over a two-year period, the hysterectomy rate decreased by half with no evident change in the community's health status. This came about not through punitive actions or reductions in reimbursement, but entirely through education and sharing of data. Importantly, there was no decrease in patient satisfaction as the rate of surgeries fell. There was a dramatic lowering of the number of complications and adverse events in each hospital as fewer patients were exposed to procedures. Costs to implement the program were minimal, consisting almost entirely of staff and physician time. The results were significant enough to interest GM in applying this process to other cities and other procedures, particularly ones that show large variation in use and indications.

Future Directions

The tidal wave of interest in reducing medical error has yet to crest. In Congress, as would be expected, a raft of legislation will be proposed over the next several years to address this public concern (*Evidence-Based Medicine*, 2000). Managed care, as this chapter has discussed, is well situated to be an important part of the ultimate solution. Health plans will be instrumental in pushing forward several key initiatives that will likely be part of the new paradigm of medical care designed to maximize patient safety.

Use of *evidence-based medicine* (EBM) will be driven by both managed care organizations and people and institutions in academic medicine, two groups that have not collaborated well in the past. EBM seeks to set objective standards for the quality of evidence that is used in the validation of medical treatments and protocols. Although the need to set such standards may seem self-evident, and a part of medicine historically, in fact EBM is a new concept. In an era when the volume of health information is growing exponentially, and when new data often contradict established tradition, it is EBM that offers the best approach for grounding care in a scientific framework so that the decisions made are of the highest quality (Booth, 2000). In EBM, treatment effects are expressed as one of several therapeutic summary measures. With these measures, one can trend care patterns more accurately, identifying deviation as it contributes to either occult failure or overt error. These measures also permit greater reproducibility in decision making, increasing the consistency sought by consumers. MCOs have taken the lead in promoting EBM by basing their medical policies on it and requiring appeals of benefit determinations to be discussed in the context of the best available scientific information.

This trend will accelerate as employers become even more involved in health benefit issues. The passivity of the 1980s is a thing of the past among employers, as demonstrated by GM's efforts in

Anderson. Managed care will be seen by these activist and sophisticated employers as a vehicle for implementing their ideas on care management. Of course, error reduction will be a prime goal. An interesting example of this new direction is the Leapfrog Group, a health issues think tank whose members are organizations that purchase health care benefits. Leapfrog is supported by the Business Roundtable (made up of the CEOs of the Fortune 200 companies). It has endorsed various initiatives and then carried them to MCOs for implementation. One such project is the use of computer-assisted pharmacy ordering in hospitals, which meshes closely with the Anthem initiative presented earlier. The group intends to use these principles as *purchasing goals* for members' employees to use as they independently decide where to spend their medical care dollars. Implementation will require collaboration between health plans and employers and individual hospitals. As the pressure from the major payers grows, augmented by the increasing concerns of their employees, managed care will devote even more resources to meeting the urgent requests of its customers to deal aggressively with patient safety issues.

Each of the initiatives mentioned is ripe for coordination with a World Wide Web option. Posting outcomes, best practices, and benchmarks on a company's Intranet for use by the employee needing care is technically feasible today. The functionality of the Internet lends itself to a host of possibilities for solving vexing aspects of error management. For example, one of the greatest challenges for providers and MCOs is eliciting reports of adverse events so that a quality improvement process can be applied. In our litigious society, few are brave enough to self-report errors. Yet without this critical feedback, recognizing process failures becomes impossible. One Internet Company, DoctorQuality.com, has begun to develop an answer to this problem. Visitors to the site can enter detailed information on sentinel events, with confidentiality assured. Data are collected, trended, and delivered back (with analysis if requested) to the provider client. This option permits quick, standardized retrieval of information in a form that is meaningful to the quality reviewer.

Each of the ideas presented here depends on bringing the patient more completely into the picture. One major change now underway due to managed care is the demise of the docile patient, content to receive instructions passively from a doctor and then to do as told. Individuals in their simultaneous roles as patient, health plan member, and employee must also function as informed consumers. MCOs have the competencies to help them achieve this new status and become not only better protected from medical error but better able to be active decision makers in their care.

Conclusion

We are on the cusp of the initiatives described in this chapter. Most are still in their initial stages, with definitive results one or two years away. The lessons from other settings, especially the aviation industry, as cited earlier, strongly support a systems focus as the best direction to pursue. MCOs are uniquely positioned to accomplish this task. No other entity collects such detailed information across virtually every site of care in a community. One impediment to success in this role is the negative perception many people have of managed care. As the health system evolves, it is to be hoped that these perceptions will change as managed care itself becomes more sophisticated in developing a medical management philosophy that is widely accepted by consumers and physicians. One way to achieve the restoration of trust in what health plans do is to deliver a method of improving patient safety and reducing iatrogenic injuries.

References

Agency for Healthcare Policy and Research. (2000, April). *Reducing errors in healthcare* (AHPQ Publication No. 00-PO58) [On-line]. Available: www.ahrq.gov/research/errors.htm

American Association of Health Plans. (1999). *1999 Industry Survey*. Washington, DC: Author.

American College of Obstetricians and Gynecologists. (1994, May). *Uterine Leiomyomata* (Technical Bulletin 192). Washington, DC: Author.

Anderson, G. F. (1997). In search of value: An international comparison of cost, access and outcomes. *Health Affairs, 16*(6), 163–171.

Bates, D. W., Teich, J. M., Lee, J., Seger, D., Kuperman, G. J., Ma'Luf, N., Boyle, D., & Leape, L. L. (1999). The impact of computerized physician order entry on medication error prevention. *Journal of the American Medical Information Association, 6*(4), 313–321.

Bazzoli, F. (2000, January). New network, new efficiencies. *Health Data Management*, pp. 32–36.

Booth, B. (2000, January 24). IOM report spurs momentum for patient safety movement. *American Medical News* [On-line]. Available: www.Ama-assn .org/sci-pubs/amnews

Duncan, W. J. (1995). *Strategic management of health care organizations*. Malden, MA: Blackwell.

Evidence-based medicine: A look at its strengths and weaknesses. (2000, January–February). (Conference Reports). *Managed Care and Cancer*, pp. 39–46.

Gross, C. P., Nicholson, W., & Powe, N. R. (1999). Factors affecting prophylactic oophorectomy in postmenopausal women. *Obstetrics and Gynecology, 94*, 962–968.

Hallam, K. (2000, January 31). Hearings look at fixes for medical errors. *Modern Healthcare*, pp. 8–9.

Kohn, L. T., Corrigan, J. M., & Donaldson, M. S. (Eds.); Committee on Quality of Health Care in America, Institute of Medicine. (2000). *To err is human: Building a safer health system*. Washington, DC: National Academy Press.

Lawrence, D. M. (2000, January 15). Managed care is not the problem. *OB GYN News*, p. 8.

Leape, L. L. (1994). Error in medicine. *Journal of the American Medical Association, 272*, 1851–1857.

Marber, S. (2000, January). Growth of CAM presents new choices, challenges for employers. *Employee Benefit News*, pp. 29–31.

McCormack, J. (2000, January). Group practices find their way to the Internet. *Health Data Management*, pp. 46–53.

McDonald, C. J. (1999). Quality measures and electronic medical systems. *Journal of the American Medical Association, 282*, 1181–1183.

Moore, J. D. (2000, January 24). One thing leads to another: Medical errors report means money for medical outcomes research. *Modern Healthcare*, pp. 2–11.

Phelps, C. E. (1992). *Health economics*. New York: HarperCollins.

Robinson, J. C. (1999). The future of managed care organization. *Health Affairs*, *18*(2), 7–24.

van Amerongen, D. (1998). *Networks and the future of medical practice*. Chicago: Health Administration Press.

7

Risk Management and Medical Errors

Margaret Copp Dawson, Ann P. Munro,
Kenneth J. Appleby, and Susan Anderson

Risk management can be an important contributor to the effort to reduce medical errors. This ability to contribute in a meaningful way to the problem of medical error is a result of the particular set of traits and skills found in risk management and the unique position risk management holds in health care organizations. This chapter sets forth the support for this assertion and calls for study to validate the usefulness of this area of activity in health care.

Risk managers possess skills in investigation, analysis, political sensitivity, and communication that are great assets in tackling any problem of this magnitude and importance. In essence they succeed as negotiators and bring this success to bear on the effort to improve patient safety. In addition, the field of risk management has traditionally employed the approach from which the quality management process of plan-do-check-act is derived: that is, analyze the problem, propose a solution, implement the solution, monitor and evaluate the solution, propose an alternative solution as indicated. The position the risk management function holds in an organization and the influence it has, which derives from its involvement in litigation and claims, places it in excellent position to be a leader in the patient safety arena. That is, risk management has credibility and is worthy of trust in the views of both clinicians and administrators. Without this trust, risk management could not function.

Although the precise degree of trust must be a subject for study by academics, as a practical matter, trust does exist and receives careful nurturing. The credibility arises from the concern risk management has for the financial health of the health care organization. Administrators see risk managers as allies in their struggles to maintain a respectable bottom line and to meet external compliance and regulatory requirements in the industry. Trust and credibility are earned on a daily basis as risk managers provide support for clinicians in dealing with difficult situations in patient care and in keeping the fear of litigation at bay.

Definition

Risk management is a profession that strives to conserve the resources of an institution, primarily financial resources, through the identification and reduction of risk and the provision of insurance programs to protect against loss. In health care, as in industry, the term *resources* is understood to include highly skilled personnel; the time and energy, both physical and emotional, of the highly skilled personnel; the physical plant and specialized equipment; and the safety of patients and employees. Protecting an institution's financial resources can be accomplished "by assuring adequate, appropriate insurance coverage against potential liability, by reducing liability when untoward events do occur, and by preventing those events that are most likely to lead to liability" (Chapman-Cliburn, 1986, p. 5).

Risk management has close working ties with or in some cases includes the medico-legal field and the arena of quality improvement.

History and Context

Risk management springs from the world of business finance. It became a separate discipline in the early twentieth century, initially in the shipping industry. The first identifiable risk manager, who also pioneered the development of the field, was a prominent French authority on general management, Henri Fayol. Around 1816, Fayol recognized *security activity* as one of six basic activities of an industrial undertaking. He stated that the object of security activity "is to safeguard property and persons against theft, fire and flood, to ward off strikes and felonies and broadly all social disturbances or natural disturbances liable to endanger the progress and even the life of the business. It is generally speaking all measures conferring security upon the undertaking and requisite peace of mind upon the personnel" (Fayol, 1949, p. 14).

Business and finance seek stability and predictability. In the 1980s, the health care industry moved closer to assuming the identity of a business operation. This shift in identity was driven by major changes, primarily limitations, in third-party reimbursement. Already, in the mid-1970s the cost of medical malpractice insurance had risen to nearly equal the cost of claims. New financing mechanisms were sought, leading to a movement toward more self-insurance and captive insurance strategies. At the same time, the cost of medical malpractice claims escalated astronomically. Risk management's role in providing stability and predictability for the business of health care gave the field new prominence.

Risk management activities are much broader in health care than they are in other industries. For example, the Michigan Society for Healthcare Risk Management (MSHRM), founded in 1979, has as its goal "better patient care through awareness and risk reduction." The American Society for Healthcare Risk Management (ASHRM), founded in 1980, defines itself as a "professional society for individuals responsible for the process of making and carrying out decisions that will promote quality care, maintain a safe environment, and safeguard financial assets." In part the mission, vision, and values of the institutions in which health care risk management operates drive such goals. ASHRM has adopted a statement of ethics, a step that is extraordinary in the overall risk management field. A large percentage of health care risk managers have come out of the health professions, primarily nursing and public health, and the views they bring with them may well influence the values that govern their new field.

Present Context

As we enter the twenty-first century, risk management is again at the center of major changes as society focuses on health care quality and patient safety. The turbulence of managed care as it assumed the majority of the health care market in the 1990s has given rise to new public sensitivity and has opened the door to greater scrutiny of health care by independent and governmental bodies. The health care industry performs *miracles* every day with rapidly advancing technology and medical treatment. This has engendered very high expectations for care among health care consumers — who are the context in which health care occurs — and little tolerance for care that deviates from near-perfect quality. The public now demands greater assurance of ideal outcomes. Indeed, the health care professions now focus on outcomes, and the two groups come together in efforts to reduce bad outcomes and eliminate injury due to human errors in the provision of health care.

The domain of risk management varies from institution to institution and depends on the size of the institution and where the risk management function is positioned in the organizational structure. Its location in the institutional structure heavily influences both its orientation and its degree of influence as a force for change. Historically, risk management has had direct ties with the financial arm of health care organizations. Since the early 1970s, health care risk management has been focused on the procurement of professional liability insurance and the management of medical malpractice claims and litigation. The driving forces for this focus have been the ever-increasing cost and limited availability of malpractice insurance, the volatility of the insurance marketplace, liberalization of the tort system, and the large financial impact of medical malpractice costs on the bottom line. Risk managers have been emphasizing for years, without much success, the importance of focusing on risk prevention and devoting resources to that process. Now, with the national focus on patient safety and error reduction at the political forefront, the *pre-loss* activities of the health care organization have taken center stage.

Today the risk manager focuses on claim and litigation management, incident reporting and data analysis, sentinel event review, crisis intervention, and day-to-day consultative advice. All these activities are directed to preserving the financial resources of an institution, but just as important, they focus on improving patient safety.

In the area of claim and litigation management, the risk manager is involved in the investigation, analysis, and resolution of claims. Risk managers work very hard to develop a relationship of trust in their organization so that incidents will be reported to them and clinicians will rely on them to resolve disputes related to dissatisfaction with care or potentially avoidable bad outcomes. Risk managers possess a particular set of skills and traits relevant to effective investigation. These include being curious, having no hidden agenda, being politically sensitive, and having good communication and analytical skills. These characteristics enable risk managers to gather facts without engendering fear or defensiveness, which can cover up rather than illuminate medical error. Skill in communicating facts in a dispassionate manner is an asset in investigating claims and transfers readily into the effort to reduce medical errors, as any analysis begins with a reconstruction of the particular chain of events and the system in which an event occurred. The importance of the risk manager's ability to establish an atmosphere in which trust is present and blame is absent cannot be overemphasized. Risk managers are negotiators. Although employed by the health care organization, the risk manager assumes a dispassionate role and advocates for each side (patient, administration or management, and clinician) in reaching a resolution satisfactory to all parties.

Gathering Information About Deviations

Developing a picture of what is happening in day-to-day operations requires knowing the systems in place and the deviations from normal operations. Information about these deviations (*incidents*, or *occurrences*) is routed to risk management through telephone and personal communications, e-mails, and incident reports. The majority of deviations reported to risk management are minor, usually involving no injury to patients. Only a small percentage result in patient harm.

Incident reporting systems typically enjoy protection from use in tort litigation and therefore provide a fairly reliable picture of what is actually happening in a given organization. Clinicians exhibit a great sense of professional responsibility in providing accurate information to the incident reporting system. Concern remains regarding the completeness of the reporting. Studies speculate that a significant portion of actual incidents are not reported (West, 2000; Serb, 1997), but it is believed that incident reporting systems obtain a representative sample. This is especially true when the incident data set includes reports from patients, nurses, social workers, and physicians as well as allegations from claims. However, increased reporting of so-called close calls or near misses will produce an even larger data set for analysis.

Gathering and analysis of the data and then reporting incident data to administration and clinical groups can provide these groups with clues about the potential for medical error and trigger studies with additional data gathering or deeper analyses of specific incidents. Incident report data can also confirm that efforts to analyze and improve a system are properly focused. To make such analysis and reporting of adverse outcomes more functional, risk managers and critics and commentators alike cite the need for a *standardized taxonomy* (Victoroff, 1997). It is thought that this would facilitate aggregate analysis and establish a cornerstone for a scientific study of medical error. Such a database would continue to need protection from journalist and litigator access.

Consider for a moment the numbers of reported incidents in a large academic medical center over a decade. Between 75 and 80 percent of the reported incidents (over 31,000) resulted in no discernable patient impact or injury. The severity of the remaining 20 percent ranged from "temporary insignificant" to "death," with the large preponderance falling into the "temporary insignificant" and "minor" categories. This certainly corroborates the conventional wisdom that approximately 20 percent of occurrences will cause 80 percent of the losses (West, 2000, p. 28). In fact, these data from a major medical center suggest that less than 10 percent of incidents reported result in 95 percent of the financial loss.

The Value of Single Event Analysis

Through the trending of incident report data and the aggregation of claims data, risk management can make a valuable contribution to the effort to reduce medical errors by raising specific issues for further study and analysis. Likewise, the careful and detailed analysis of a single untoward event can lead to the detection of critical issues and system flaws. Consider the following example: a patient experiences a complication from a procedure. She asserts a claim for medical costs, economic or wage loss, and pain and suffering, plus loss of consortium by her husband. Risk management undertakes an investigation. Review by a committee of the medical staff, a regular part of the claim resolution process, occurs. This triggers a review of the complication rate for this procedure. It is determined that significant variation exists in how and by whom the procedure is performed. This information is relayed to the Quality Management Committee, which conducts an internal review and contracts with an outside reviewer to compare complication rates and processes. The result is a redefinition of privileges, which reduces variation in the process. Monitoring by the quality management function follows to determine whether the solution indeed fixed the problem and whether the correction remains in place. The required review of sentinel events for the Joint Commission for Accreditation of Healthcare Organizations (JCAHO) takes similar advantage of the intense analysis of a single event to draw common causes and produce systemwide improvements. This process, driven by risk management in coordination with quality management, can be fruitful in developing improvements in clinical care that have clinician buy-in because they flow from actual experience and are based initially on clinician review and opinion.

Sentinel Events

In 1999, JCAHO began to require each organization it accredits to have in place a policy and a process to address *sentinel events* that occur in the organization. The process includes the reporting of the event, an investigation, a root cause analysis and development of corrective action to address the root causes, implementation of an action plan, and ongoing monitoring to ensure that changes made remain in place. Many health care organizations had such a formal or informal process in place earlier in the 1990s. The JCAHO requirement raised the visibility of the existing policies and underscored for all staff their institutional importance.

Risk management provides important leadership in this process in many institutions and has full responsibility for it in others, often working closely with quality improvement efforts in the analysis and implementation stages. Monitoring implemented changes for effectiveness in reducing the likelihood of error recurrence falls most commonly in the area of quality improvement. Sentinel events, which by definition are the result of errors or flaws in some system for the provision of health care, are important opportunities for analysis of both proximate and common causes. The *proximate cause* is understood as the specific cause of the single event under analysis. *Common causes* are those that are revealed in the course of reviewing a specific event but that may have broader implications throughout the particular organization and over time. Lessons learned in reviewing sentinel events are communicated by the JCAHO to other health care organizations, often through the risk managers, whose national organization, ASHRM, works cooperatively with

JCAHO for the responsible analysis of medical errors. In this case, an external force (namely JCAHO) supports the values and intentions of not only risk management but also the rest of the organization, administrative and clinical, in improving quality of patient care.

Systems that serve to protect patients make good use of risk management data, analysis, and investigative skills. These systems include the process to credential and privilege physicians and to credential and privilege other clinicians in expanded roles (nurse practitioners, physician's assistants, and nurse anesthetists, for example), quality assurance programs, and compliance activities. Gathering data concerning physicians' claim and litigation history and, more important, interpreting these data makes good use of risk managers' expertise. Likewise, data gathered in risk management incident-reporting systems provide a basis for quality assurance activities that monitor changes and illuminate trends and areas for focused study. Health care organizations rely on the assistance of risk managers in compliance activities and in responding to external regulatory bodies. Risk managers regularly interact with regulatory organizations including accrediting bodies (JCAHO and the National Committee on Quality Assurance), licensing agencies, and federal government agencies such as the Food and Drug Administration. Issues that arise in this arena provide important information for proactive change; in this capacity risk management serves as a conduit for information between the agency and the organization. For example, the Safe Medical Device Act requires organizations to report patient injury related to medical devices to the FDA so that national data can be aggregated and potential risks to patients eliminated. Risk management may investigate cases of patient injury and may participate in the evaluation of events reported within the organization and then reported to the federal government.

Risk managers as a rule have an interest in developing their image as helpful advocates for both clinicians and patients as well as for the administrative structure to which they belong. They often find themselves in the role of consultants to clinicians and patients on the wide variety of issues that can arise as all parties attempt to negotiate a path through a complex organizational process and structure. Again, communication skills and abilities to gather pertinent facts and to define issues in difficult, sometimes-contentious situations enable risk managers to render an important service to health care staff and to patients. This reinforces a relationship of trust, which supports quality improvement efforts to analyze systems in order to reduce medical errors. The analytical skills at play in this day-to-day work to define problems transfer into the medical error arena with great success.

Support for clinical staff in handling troublesome situations, investigation and follow-up of adverse and sentinel events, participation in credentialing and privileging activities, and involvement with safety, compliance, and quality improvement all lie within the domain of risk management in a health care organization. What should be obvious is that each of these areas offers opportunities for reducing injury due to medical errors. Property loss, workers' compensation programs, general liability claims, and patient relations may also fall under the umbrella of risk management, although these activities are less directly related to the provision of health care services.

Models of Risk Management

The form that risk management takes in a given organization may vary considerably. The primary determinants of that form are the duties or areas of responsibility that make up the risk management domain and the way risk management fits into the organizational reporting structure.

Having responsibility for insurance procurement or reporting through the finance function can shift the focus of risk management away from clinical issues, despite recognition of the importance of proactive response to those issues. Conversely, close ties with finance give recommendations from risk management a stronger impact in forcing organizational change and in obtaining dollars to make changes toward more consistent, higher-quality patient care. In this arrangement, the quality management effort may drive the analysis and recommendations, with the influence of risk management encouraging change.

Having some responsibility for claims and litigation or reporting through the legal structure provides risk management with similar armaments in the arena of change for quality patient care. Sensitivity to the cost of medical errors that result in significant patient injury and wind up in litigation or in informal resolution arises from involvement in this area. In addition, credibility attaches to this involvement, increasing risk management's power of persuasion in implementing change.

One danger of a close alliance between risk management and the legal or claims structures is that changes that affect the quality of care but do not address areas in which high-cost claims arise may be given less attention or less importance among the many issues begging for the scarce resources of time and money.

Yet another structure in which risk management may be found is the clinical structure. If this is a powerful force in the organization—if it is, for example, the physician leadership structure—then the impact risk management has on clinical care is enhanced. Agreed-on changes in clinical practice are more readily and systematically implemented. If risk management is aligned with a less powerful group, such as nursing, its impact and influence are diminished.

Large medical centers and health systems often centralize and divide risk management duties. The insurance procurement functions may reside in finance and be separate from the clinical risk functions. There may be a separate legal office that handles formal claims and litigation in addition to other legal concerns of the business enterprise of health care. On-site risk managers may handle the day-to-day events and complaints, field calls from clinicians, and work closely with quality management to tease out issues relevant for study. Finance and legal risk management may rely heavily on the information and analysis garnered by clinical risk management about individual and aggregated claims, incidents, and investigations.

Smaller community hospitals generally combine risk management functions with a related area, as described previously, or with medical records, nursing, or the office of the CEO. These combination arrangements present major challenges in developing focus and expertise in analysis. In addition, the relationship of trust with clinicians, which is essential to good risk management, may be eroded by the potential conflict in roles. For example, when one person is both investigating an incident and dealing with any disciplinary action that may arise from the incident, the truthfulness of the information received during the investigation may be in doubt.

Finally, investigation and claims handling as well as litigation management may be contracted to consulting and claims management firms or to specialists retained by the insurance company. In this arrangement, ensuring good feedback to the quality management group is a significant challenge, as the focus is less on proactive involvement in error reduction than on the swift and economical resolution of the claim.

Assets

Within any organization, risk management has no authority except over its own operations. The influence risk management brings to any process, including the change process, is just that: the power of persuasion, though based on sound data and reasoning.

Key to the maintenance of this influence is perceived neutrality. Risk management has no agenda of its own save better patient care and the financial health of its organization. It is vulnerable to being pulled into struggles for scarce resources and must be wary of efforts to involve it in the political battles in the organization. Risk managers are challenged to remain above personal and personality conflicts and competition, not allowing their own feelings or alliances to dictate or even guide their analyses and recommendations. Conversely, risk managers can have influence on the institutional view and vision. Risk management can play a major role in establishing an organizational climate that supports truth telling, both internally and to patients. This greatly facilitates the flow of information that is critical to meaningful process improvement, and supports the sense of trust and *right mission* that encourages clinician participation. Discretion, diplomacy, and confidentiality are qualities associated with good risk management operations. Risk managers can rely on institutional mission and vision statements, professional statements of ethics, and their own code of ethics to guide them through difficult conflicts. Risk management is often perceived to wield considerable power in an organization. It is, however, the power of influence, not authority, carefully nurtured and maintained.

Barriers

A major barrier to successful analysis and improvement in health care, in addition to the massive complexity of health care organizations, is the existence of cultural subgroups within that complex system. These subgroups often experience great difficulty in communicating with each other. They may not share a common view of a particular process or problem, let alone a common goal for its improvement or resolution. This barrier may prevent fruitful discussions or truthful raising of issues. This is particularly the case when there is competition for resources, when budget pressures are great, or when there is a perceived power differential or territorial conflict. For example, surgeons and the administration might tangle over the purchase of new, expensive equipment or devices; nursing might battle with the administration for an increased budget for overtime when the patient load is especially heavy or when additional staff time is taken up by training to keep up with changes in technology. In both cases, each group might try to gain the support of risk management for its position. In response, risk management's best course of action is to raise legitimate issues of patient safety and quality of care, raise questions of relative risk and benefit, and avoid taking a stand on any particular outcome.

Risk management can employ its communication skills and exploit its perceived neutrality by acting as a bridge between competing groups or between different cultures: surgeons and internists, for example, or doctors and nurses, or pharmacists and everyone else.

Consider the senior internist who discounts a nurse's perceptions and discourages transmission of information about changes in a patient's condition but is also known for strong negative reactions to being disturbed during a meeting or rounds, the anesthesiologists who complain that a surgeon shuts down communication during a case, or the surgeon who complains that anesthesiologists don't communicate critical patient data. In all three cases, patient safety is at risk, and risk management may be called upon to referee the discussion, sometimes through the use of a process especially designed for multidisciplinary review of difficult cases and poor outcomes.

Inadequate, inaccurate, incomplete, or unintelligible communication and false assumptions (failures to communicate) pose enormous risks to patient safety in a system that depends on teamwork for the smooth coordination of complex care.

Limitations

Serious limitations exist in what we can learn from our data, and caution in drawing conclusions without focused study is warranted. Aggregate data offer an opportunity to view events throughout a health care organization or system. Comparisons made through benchmarking with other bodies can illuminate issues, as can trending the data over time. Significant limitations exist, however, sounding a note of caution to those who would base analysis of medical error on data alone. Here are important issues to be considered:

- What is the quality of the data derived from self-reporting? For example: what percentage of events is actually reported? do competing agendas (such as professional duty, an interest in a different resource allocation, or a concern for making a particular systemic change (such as authorizing additional staff or overtime or altering a system of medication delivery) influence what is brought forward?

- Do errors, events, or incidents that do not result in patient injury, tell us anything important? Where should we direct our resources? This is a critical question.

- Are data accumulated from a system of self-reporting valid? Studies have been conducted that compare reported incidents to events recorded concurrently in medical records. Incident reports can be compared concurrently or retrospectively with incidents witnessed by trained observers using hospital-based ethnographic methodology.

- What conclusions can be drawn? Can conclusions be drawn from valid data and compared to benchmark data with denominators that allow a rate to be established? Further research may assist an organization to develop methods and criteria for using specific data in ways other than further intense study of a particular issue. All resources in the health care industry are scarce, including those directed toward the scrutiny of systems.

- For what purpose will data be used? An obvious barrier to obtaining complete data is concern that information and documents generated in sincere efforts to improve quality and reduce medical errors may be used to support the plaintiff's case in a litigated claim. The potential financial implications of this risk are enormous.

- To what extent are data timely? In an era of rapid and accelerating change, the timeliness of data on which any analysis, including systems analysis, is based is important in determining the merit of a particular conclusion. An analysis of a closed case (a resolved claim, whether litigated or not) offers the benefit of outside review of an event with a negative patient outcome, but closed cases are usually not available for analysis until three to five years after the event, not close enough to the actual event to permit timely analysis of the system involved. More useful is the professional judgment contained in the outside expert review. This judgment may be useful for directing subsequent training and education, particularly if information from a systems analysis conducted in the initial risk management investigation can also be applied.

- How comprehensive are the available analytical tools? Can they effectively embrace the complexity of the health care system — or its parts?

- Is size important? The size of an organization does not necessarily correlate with the effectiveness or sophistication of risk management and that function's role in reducing medical errors.

Past Disappointments and Failures

Risk management has a core of concern for the patient, yet it has fiscal responsibility as its foremost charge. It is bound by concern for the costs of professional liability claims. This concern is both advantageous and disadvantageous for the change process. The U.S. tort system, touted by many as a driving force in health care improvement, may indeed propel a health care organization or individual clinicians to embrace change in an effort to avoid financial disaster. There may be some truth to the notion that fear of litigation is one force driving improvements geared to reduce patient injury. However, the quality of such change is severely limited by the dampening effect the tort system has on the free flow of information and exchange of ideas. Although bona fide quality improvement documents enjoy statutory protection from discovery in many states, there remains genuine concern that certain information may be damaging to a case even if the documents that substantiate it are protected.

Perhaps the greatest negative impact of the present tort system on quality improvement is the caution it arouses in health care organizations when it comes to sharing information regionally and nationally. Even within an organization and even given statutory protection, there may be hesitation to discuss lessons learned with large groups for fear that information may be distorted and shared with potential adversaries. Litigation is very serious to institutions and clinicians. Careers can be ruined, personal lives destroyed or severely damaged. Defensive changes in practice that are not cost effective may be imposed in response to the fear of litigation. Of greatest importance, however, is the dampening of free and open discussion of patient outcomes that are less than desired.

The lens of litigation is always retrospective and therefore subject to hindsight bias. Even the expert opinions obtained by the opposing sides in a lawsuit are not true peer review. They are obtained deliberately to bolster one point of view or the other and are based not on information current with the contested event but on knowing the end of the story. Once you know what was found at autopsy, for example, it is easy to look back and say that a particular diagnosis was obvious. The daily practice of medicine, however, is based on probabilities, not on certainties. Although quality improvement recognizes this premise and takes it into account in analyzing processes and outcomes, the litigation system remains blind to it.

Litigation is driven by bad outcomes and is based on the premise that bad outcomes are the result of malpractice, because this is the standard for compensation in our present system. Fault is found and individuals blamed. All bad outcomes are not the result of medical errors, yet our system for compensation does not acknowledge this. In the legal arena, different parties with vested interests in the outcome of the analysis, and using different standards, come to the table. This process contributes little to the reduction of error and improved patient outcomes.

Future Possibilities

Risk management has the potential to take a leadership role, in partnership with clinical staff and quality improvement efforts, in the systematic reduction of medical errors and enhancement of quality in health care in the United States. Tort reform can also play a significant role. Some argue that if we are serious about reducing medical errors, we should adopt a system of enterprise liability in order to remove the faultfinding and avoid the diversion of scarce health care dollars and energy from the true mission of the health care system — the provision of care.

Risk management can become the locus of systems analysis expertise, bringing the useful tool of systems analysis to bear on the almost infinitely complex health care delivery system, teasing apart the pieces of the system and bringing enlightenment where there was once confusion. At the same time, care must be taken to avoid oversimplification, as might occur in an overly literal adoption of the systems analysis that has been successful in, for example, the airline industry. Risk managers are challenged to develop expertise in this area and to bring to the efforts to reduce medical errors the best thinking in other fields, applying this thinking wisely.

Risk management can do much to promote a climate of truth telling and bolster the current willingness to confront the realities within health care systems. Only from this basis can real improvement proceed. The human factor in health care — the emotional commitment of health care professionals and their willingness to bring the very essence of their person to the care of patients—cannot be ignored. To injure a patient through error can be devastating to a health care professional or caregiver. Those professionals and caregivers who become victims themselves of imperfect systems and inadvertently inflict harm must be supported. Their attempts to name the problem, to correct the flaws, must be respected. Their safety, too, is the responsibility of all engaged in this endeavor.

Efforts to reduce the financial pressures on health systems must continue, as this is essential to support system changes. Because we cannot return to the free spending of the sixties and seventies, society must grapple with the difficult issues of access to health care and the development of rational use criteria for limited resources. Control over runaway *technolust* (if a high-tech process can be done it must be a good thing and must be implemented wherever possible) must be maintained.

Conclusion

Clearly there is great untapped potential for addressing medical errors and flaws in our health care system in general. Our challenges are how to apply the best thinking in systems analysis, how to obtain and interpret data, how to implement change, and how to care for caregivers as well as the patients. We have the knowledge to provide excellent health care for our population. Certainly the population expects to receive this type of care. We can name the problems and the barriers and address them. Risk management can offer unique contributions to this effort.

References

Chapman-Cliburn, G. (Ed.). (1986). *Risk management and quality assurance issues and interactions* (Special publication of the *Quality Review Bulletin*). Chicago: Joint Commission on Accreditation of Hospitals.

Fayol, H. (1949). *General and industrial management.* New York: Pitman.

Serb, C. (1997, July 5). The uncalculated risks: Why risk managers won't benchmark. *Hospitals & Health Networks, 71*(13), 28–30.

Victoroff, M. S. (1997, July). The right intentions: Errors and accountability [Editorial]. *The Journal of Family Practice, 45,* 38–39.

West, J. C. (2000). Comparing risk management information: An invitation to disaster. *Journal of Healthcare Risk Management, 20*(1), 20–30.

8

Can Evidence-Based Medicine and Outcomes Research Contribute to Error Reduction?

Susan D. Horn, Joanne V. Hickey,
Theresa L. Carroll, and Anne-Claire I. France

Few reports have generated as much concern about the fundamental quality of health care in the United States as *To Err Is Human: Building a Safer Health System* (Kohn, Corrigan, & Donaldson, 2000). This Institute of Medicine (IOM) report estimates that 98,000 people die each year from medical errors that occur in hospitals, and asserts that the problem is not bad people in health care but good people who are using bad systems that need to be made safer. The report sets out a national agenda to reduce medical errors and improve patient safety through a safer health system. The federal task force created to address medical errors after the IOM report was published is recommending mandatory reporting, the specifics of which are to be determined. As a result, many researchers have begun an urgent search for strategies to prevent medical errors and rebuild confidence in the system. Although there is some controversy about the IOM findings, all will agree that patients will benefit if errors are reduced (McDonald, Weiner, & Hui, 2000; Leape, 2000).

Outcomes research provides a scientific way to examine patient outcomes and determine best practices in delivering care. Thus *evidence-based medicine* and outcomes research offer a means to examine and evaluate practices related to care. Once potential problems and system or organizational factors associated with errors have been identified from scientific data, clinicians can replace dangerous practices with redesigned practices that reduce medical errors. Specifically, once one discovers which systems or practices at the organizational level and which treatments and processes at the patient level are associated with better outcomes and fewer errors, one can institute those systems, treatments, and processes, with the result that the quality of care is improved.

We believe that better outcomes and error reduction can be achieved through the use of a new multidimensional outcomes methodology called *clinical practice improvement* (CPI). CPI methodology can examine and address the contribution to medical errors and patient safety made both by organizational or systems factors and by individual patient treatments. We explain how in the remainder of this chapter.

In this discussion, we adopt the Institute of Medicine definition of a medical error: "the failure of a planned action to be completed as intended or the use of a wrong plan to achieve an aim," whether or not the error results in harm (pp. 4, 28). It is natural to consider whether such medical errors can be reduced through more careful attention to evidence-based medicine (EBM), an approach in which medical decisions involve the judicious identification, evaluation, and application of practice-based evidence and the strength of that evidence. It is clearly important to evaluate the strength of evidence from both basic scientific and patient-centered clinical research. Patient-centered clinical research focuses on such clinically relevant areas as the accuracy and precision of diagnostics; the power of prognostic markers; and the efficacy and safety of therapeutic, rehabilitation, and preventive regimens. It has been estimated that strong scientific evidence exists for only about 15 percent of common health care practices (Williamson, Goldschmidt, & Jillson, 1979). Yet, patients do need care, and treatment decisions must be made based on available knowledge and *best practice*. Best practice is a combination of available EBM, consensus reports, clinician's judgment, and patient preference.

The Evidence for Evidence-Based Medicine

The research base for EBM spans a range of elements from the Cochrane Collaboration methodology to clinical guidelines (see Figure 8.1).

The Cochrane Collaboration is a worldwide network of participants who attempt to follow a standard for review of relevant literature on a specific topic, such as drug therapy for stage II heart failure (Altman & Burton, 1999). Only randomized controlled trials (RCTs) are reviewed, and only RCTs that meet specific standards and make what is thought to be an important scientific contribution are summarized. Cochrane collaborators report a meta-analysis of pertinent studies on a topic, with an indication of the strength of the findings for practice.

Individually and locally developed guidelines or protocols may have little organized scientific basis and often represent the opinions of the author or of a small group. Outcomes research examines differences in outcomes but does not relate those outcomes to detailed patient characteristics or treatment or process differences under a clinician's control. The multidimensional clinical practice improvement methodology is a type of outcomes research that measures detailed patient severity and other patient characteristics, detailed treatment and process steps, and patient outcomes and

Cochrane Collaboration
    Randomized controlled trials
        Clinical practice improvement/multidimensional CPI
            Quasi-experimental studies
            Outcomes research
                Consensus expert panel reports
                    Expert panel guidelines/protocols
                        Guidelines/protocols generated
                        by individuals/local groups

Figure 8.1. Range of Evidence for Clinical Practice.

attempts to identify meaningful associations of input variables with outcomes.

Regardless of the strength of scientific evidence and the research foundation of the evidence, external clinical evidence can inform, but can never replace, individual clinical expertise and judgment. The expert clinician must determine whether the external evidence applies to the individual patient, and if it does, how it should be applied to a clinical decision and patient care.

Clinical Practice Improvement Study Design

Clinical practice improvement is a new multidimensional outcomes methodology that has direct application to the clinical management of individual patients. Clinicians in actual practice create a large database of detailed patient and treatment or process variables that are important to the particular problem under study and that reflect the complexity of clinical practice and the multiple variables that affect patient outcomes. Multivariate statistical techniques identify clinically relevant relationships that explain complex clinical phenomena. CPI inquiry is multidisciplinary, involving many different types of clinicians who participate in posing clinically relevant questions, determining what variables will be identified for measurement, and implementing decisions about the treatment and care process based on the data. Clinicians who treat patients develop the definitions of all the study variables so they understand exactly how to change their practice as a result of the study findings. The multidimensional CPI methodology can also be applied to the study and identification of complex relationships of variables at the systems or organizational level.

Several aspects of the CPI approach make it attractive to clinicians who are interested in finding ways to improve patient care. First, it is a scientifically "bottom-up" approach: clinicians drive the study and determine what outcomes, treatments, and patient data are needed to describe all the relevant input and output variables. CPI helps clinicians make their own decisions about optimal care, basing those decisions on objective statistical evidence gathered in the routine, everyday practice of medicine.

Second, CPI methodology encompasses a comprehensive view of the complex care process. By collecting and analyzing measures of patient differences (for example, the physiological severity of illness and psychosocial abnormalities presented at each visit or at each admission), care process steps (that is, all treatments that are part of the care process for that condition), and outcome variables, clinicians can evaluate objectively the effects of the treatments they give to similarly ill patients. If they do not have all three types of data (for example, if they have process and outcome data but not detailed patient data), clinicians cannot tell whether the outcomes achieved are due to the process steps or to differences in patient severity levels (see Figure 8.2).

Third, the CPI methodology focuses on application. It spotlights care-related variables that can be implemented to improve outcomes. This focus on implementation guides who is involved in the design, what data are collected, what questions are answered during analyses, who interprets the findings, and who translates those findings into revised or new alterations in practice to reduce errors and improve outcomes. Measurement is repeated to confirm that

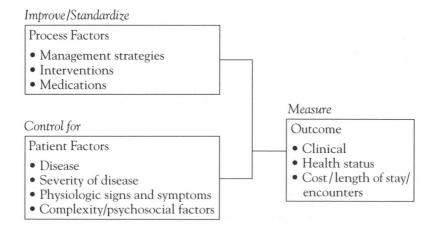

Improve/Standardize

Process Factors

- Management strategies
- Interventions
- Medications

Control for

Patient Factors

- Disease
- Severity of disease
- Physiologic signs and symptoms
- Complexity/psychosocial factors

Measure

Outcome

- Clinical
- Health status
- Cost/length of stay/ encounters

Figure 8.2. Three Essential Components for a Clinical Practice Improvement Study.

the change in practice has actually occurred and that it is associated with the desired outcome. These elements, so attractive to clinicians interested in patient-level change and improvements, can also be important to improving results at the organizational level.

Dimensions in a Clinical Practice Improvement Study Design

Many variables can be considered in each of the three essential components of a CPI study.

Patient Variables

Patient variables are the key characteristics of the population: demographics, specific indications for treatment and severity of illness, psychosocial factors, and so forth. In a well-defined, similarly ill patient group, one would expect that care processes of equal effectiveness would result in similar outcomes. For clinicians to agree to stabilize their processes of care, one needs sufficient detail describing patients and their needs, and that detail usually requires disease-specific physiological data, such as those contained in the inpatient and outpatient components of the Comprehensive Severity Index (CSI®) (Horn, 1995, 1997; Horn, Sharkey, & Levy, 1995; Horn, Sharkey, Tracy, et al., 1996; Horn, Sharkey, & Gassaway, 1996; Horn, Buckle, & Carver, 1988; Horn, Sharkey, Buckle, et al., 1991; Averill et al., 1992; Iezzoni, 1998). Detailed physiological severity data are needed to create decidable and executable treatment protocols that are based on patient signs and symptoms.

Medical Care Process Variables

A *process of care* is a set of sequentially linked steps designed to produce a set of desired medical outcomes. The goal is to find a measurable variable that describes each major process step. Examples include which drugs are dispensed, what dose is used, what route and duration of administration are chosen, how often prescriptions are filled, what ventilator settings are used, and so on. Timing data are also collected for all process steps.

Outcome Variables

Processes of care should be designed to achieve specific patient outcomes. Among the outcomes commonly assessed are diagnosis-specific complications, adverse events, diagnosis-specific long-term medical outcomes (which may be assessed by both clinicians and patients), patient functional status, patient satisfaction, and cost. Outcomes may be thought of as analogs of the assessment endpoints in a randomized controlled trial.

Analytical Methods

A CPI study database typically includes a great many variables that describe patient characteristics, processes of care, and patient outcomes. When more than three or four patient and process (independent) variables must be taken into account, multiple regression analysis is used to model the effects of these factors on the outcome (dependent) variables. Multivariate statistical methods allow comparisons of alternative treatments while controlling for other variables that may be driving observed differences between the outcomes of the treatments. These statistical methods allow the researcher to examine relationships far more complex than those defined using only one or two explanatory variables at a time. The coefficients of the independent variables in the regression equations identify key process steps that, when controlling for patient factors, are associated with better outcomes.

Clinical Practice Improvement Goes Beyond Outcomes Research

Outcomes research typically uses large, existing claims databases to find better and worse outcomes and also outcome failures (poor outcomes beyond some statistical threshold) such as high mortality rates. But most outcomes research does not lead to practice improvement or fewer errors in medicine because

- Outcome failures are not scientifically related to detailed process steps that are under a practitioner's control, so it is unclear how to improve the outcome.

- Patients are described only by diagnosis codes, so severity of illness is not controlled for.

In addition, concerns about the completeness, accuracy, and relevance of large claims databases raise questions about their appropriateness as a basis for health services research, performance monitoring (including identification and reduction of medical errors), or inspiring changes in clinical practice. A fundamental problem exists with outcomes data: data collected for one purpose (for example, claims administration) may not be useful for other purposes (for example, outcomes research) when they lack reliable, detailed information about patient differences and medical care processes.

Clinical Practice Improvement Goes Beyond Guidelines

It has been suggested that clinical guidelines be used to reduce errors in medicine. However, because most clinical practices have no firm basis in published scientific research, developers of clinical guidelines often resort to expert consensus, which is an inexact tool even when generated with formal methods. Different consensus groups have different goals and use different techniques, often developing different, even conflicting, guidelines on the same topic (Kellie & Kelly, 1991; Audet, Greenfield, & Field, 1990; Leape, Park, Kahan, & Brook, 1992). Within a single consensus panel, the experts often disagree, and their assessments change when guidelines developed in a theoretical setting are applied to real patients (Park et al., 1989). Perhaps most troubling, physician experts show wide disagreements when they assess underlying probabilities essential to consensus judgments (Eddy, 1992, 1984; O'Connor et al., 1988).

Most efforts to develop guidelines are characterized by two weaknesses that hamper the guidelines' relevance to local practice reform:

- Guidelines are developed nationally or centrally, based on expert consensus and literature review and synthesis.

- Guidelines are often too general or inconclusive to be useful to clinicians and do not address subgroups within a sample.

Thus clinicians are unwilling to follow many current guidelines.

At present evidence-based methods of guideline development are favored over consensus-based methods. However, the patient populations in which the "evidence" is gathered (usually in randomized controlled trials) are often different from those in which local translations of the guideline will be used. Because evidence-based guidelines must be all things to all people, they are often encyclopedic and equivocal. They are not decidable and executable and frequently do not have credibility with local clinicians.

Clinical Practice Improvement Differs from Randomized Controlled Trials

The randomized controlled trial has a long history as the gold standard for establishing causality in scientific research. Randomization to diminish potential selection bias and strict control of the intervention of interest are important tools for scientists of all types. However, the use of RCTs has been limited in some domains of inquiry because of such problems as these:

- Ethical or practical inability to randomize patients or to control the specificity of the intervention to be studied.

- Prohibitive cost when cell sizes or samples are extremely large.

- Exclusion of large numbers of individuals who do not meet strict inclusion criteria. Because one does not want the study outcome to be influenced by extraneous factors, patients with secondary problems or more severe disease are often rejected as subjects. Only a small percentage of patients—usually 10 to 15 percent—are typically eligible for a trial. The idea is to eliminate all patients whose characteristics might adversely affect or bias the outcome of the comparison between the treatment and the control arms.

- Potential selection bias from patient or health plan nonparticipation in studies where a limited benefit for those patients or health plans can be identified prospectively.

The alternative study designs used in clinical practice improvement offer a pragmatic balance of study cost, clinician participation, rapid patient accrual, and the need for timely information with potential bias. Achieving this balance is especially important when examining operational process-of-care factors (in contrast to testing new treatments) and when permanent data collection systems routinely track patient and process factors so that invalid inferences are likely to be found and corrected over time.

RCTs use a protocol document to create an artificial practice environment that allows valid statistical inference. Although that structure eliminates practice variation, it usually covers a very limited subset of patients and practices. CPI addresses the same issues — practice variation and valid statistical inference —from another point of view. It measures process variation, then eliminates it through a combination of statistical analysis, consensus, and feedback. Under a CPI protocol, valid statistical inference is possible because groups of similar patients receive the same treatment. RCTs also tend to be limited in time; in most circumstances, they explicitly modify clinician behavior only for the duration of a study and only for the individuals directly involved in the trial. In contrast, CPI establishes a permanent feedback loop aimed at all clinicians in an institution. It integrates research into daily practice, giving individual clinicians the information necessary to understand and modify their own activities at a detailed, operational level. CPI analyses help providers evaluate current practices and use the results to develop fact-based improvements that rest on clinical data rather than on clinical opinion.

Measuring severity and controlling for confounding variables across multiple domains permits identification of associations rather than causality; however, study of the results of sensitivity analyses and the concurrence of findings with other research can help clinicians determine whether the identified associations are real and are relevant to existing practices (Magi, Douglas, & Schwartz, 1996; Pestotnik, Classen, Evans, & Burke, 1996). Finally, because data are gathered from existing patient records, the clinical practice improvement study design has an inherently low rate of patient attrition over time, so it avoids what is a persistent problem with RCTs in health services research.

Advantages of Clinical Practice Improvement Methodology

A key advantage of clinical practice improvement methodology is the naturalistic view of medical treatment provided by retrospective data recorded routinely by medical providers. This view is critical to determining the implications of treatment alternatives. In everyday practice, patients are assigned to different treatments based on the provider's medical judgment, patient compliance is not artificially influenced, and monitoring of results is based on the provider's need for information about how a patient is doing. All these factors can affect the effectiveness of medical treatment.

This retrospective view is in direct contrast to the view obtained during traditional randomized controlled trials. Because their participants are screened, selected, and subjected to scrutiny and intervention beyond that occurring in everyday treatment, RCTs sometimes report results that are not broadly applicable in everyday medical treatment.

A second key advantage of CPI study methodology is cost. Using existing data from medical records and computerized databases is generally much less costly than implementing a prospective RCT. Other advantages of employing retrospective data include the large number of observations often available for analysis and the usefulness of the data for hypothesis generation and refinement. Observational studies do not scientifically prove the causality of any underlying relationships, but they can point to hypotheses that can be clinically evaluated. For example, application of the CPI methodology in adult patients undergoing abdominal surgery resulted in a decrease in length of hospital stay of more than 1.5 days for bowel surgery patients and more than 2.0 days for appendectomy patients, less increase in severity of illness during hospitalization, and a calculated decrease in cost of $4,000 per patient. In a separate study, CPI methodology resulted in the prevention of pressure ulcers at a rate of 302 per year and $1,268,400 in cost savings per year. Similar improved outcomes occurred when CPI methodology was used to implement guidelines for the use of heparin in adult patients with deep vein thrombosis (Horn, 1997). Recent literature has supported the use of well-designed observational studies such as CPI to discover what works best in medicine. Two studies found that treatment effects from observational studies and randomized controlled trials were remarkably similar (Benson & Hartz, 2000; Concato, Shah, & Horwitz, 2000). Both studies concluded that they found little evidence that estimates of treatment effects in well-designed observational studies were either consistently larger than or qualitatively different from those obtained in randomized controlled trials.

Multidimensional CPI Applied to Organizational Variables

We have described how CPI studies work when applied at the patient level (that is, the patient is the unit of analysis) to discover best treatments and processes for specified patient types. However, the same methodology can be used at the systems or organizational level to discover which systems or organizational characteristics, controlling for patient differences, result in the fewest number of medical errors. One can draw on the scientific work of safety-oriented industries to understand sources of error in human performance and systems operations. By analyzing systems, one can uncover latent conditions or steps in a system that lead directly to adverse events. These conditions and steps include not only processes but also human factors such as habit, cognition, fatigue, culture, attitudes, and bureaucracy.

To discover which systems approaches are best, organizations need data on how the systems are working at present, controlling for the types of patients that are treated. In order to gather these data, organizations must have the clinicians treating patients describe the situations where errors have occurred or have the potential to occur, and legislation to protect the confidentiality of certain information must be in place; for example, data on medical mistakes that have no serious consequences should be protected if they are collected and analyzed solely for the purpose of improving safety and quality. If individuals face serious consequences for reporting mistakes, even when those mistakes have no serious medical consequences, there will be less information available for the organization to analyze to discover which systems best prevent medical errors.

The best systems approaches to reducing medical errors fall into two categories: (1) short-term systems changes, those needing only a little time in which to implement the best practice, and

(2) long-term systems changes, such as those needing more thorough study or greater investment.

Examples of short-term changes include implementing proven medication safety practices, such as using automated drug-ordering systems and eliminating the similar-sounding drug names and the confusing labels and packaging that foster medication mistakes. An alternative to the latter suggestion is to place warning labels on packages of drugs with similar names. A CPI study could discover which of these approaches is associated with the fewest medication errors; after changes have been made, the system can be remeasured to determine whether the desired results have been achieved.

A CPI study conducted at the patient level requires a multidisciplinary study team that comprises all the provider types that treat patients with the specified condition. This team defines the relevant variables and assists in their analysis. Likewise, a multidimensional CPI study conducted at the systems or organizational level should consider all the parts of the health care enterprise that are involved with the product line to be studied; the people involved in each part should define their practices and assist in asking questions for practice analysis and association with best outcomes.

Conclusion

Evidence-based medicine and outcomes research using CPI provide an excellent, comprehensive, multidimensional approach to error reduction. Both methodologies use judicious identification and detailed evaluation. Combined, they can evaluate the impact of a practice and the association of all the variables pertinent to that practice with the outcomes. Because of the thorough analysis of all possible confounding factors, clinicians feel confident in using the resulting findings to guide their future clinical decisions.

Errors are often the result of a sequence of events that occurs because poorly designed systems make it difficult to detect errors and opportunities for errors (Perrow, 1984). Even simple tasks (for example, ordering a medication for a patient) often involve multiple steps, each presenting an opportunity for error.

The two primary objectives for designers of systems are (1) to make it difficult for individuals to make errors and (2) to facilitate error detection and correction before harm occurs (Leape et al., 1995). Combining evidence-based medicine and multidimensional CPI makes it possible to identify many points in systems where errors can occur and (using multivariate analyses) to determine which are associated with higher or lower error rates.

References

Altman, D. G., & Burton, M. J. (1999, October). The Cochrane Collaboration. *Langenbecks Archives of Surgery, 384*(5), 432–436.

Audet, A. M., Greenfield, S., & Field, M. (1990). Medical practice guidelines: Current activities and future directions. *Annals of Internal Medicine, 113*(9), 709–714.

Averill, R. F., McGuire, T. E., Manning, B. E., Fowler, D. A., Horn, S. D., Dickson, P. S., Coye, M. J., Knowlton, D. L., & Bender, J. A. (1992). A study of the relationship between severity of illness and hospital cost in New Jersey hospitals. *Health Services Research, 27*(5), 587–617.

Benson, K., & Hartz, A. J. (2000). A comparison of observational studies and randomized, controlled trials. *New England Journal of Medicine, 342*(25), 1878–1886.

Concato, J., Shah, N., & Horwitz, R. I. (2000). Randomized, controlled trials, observational studies, and the hierarchy of research designs. *New England Journal of Medicine, 342*(25), 1887–1892.

Eddy, D. M. (1984). Variations in physician practice: The role of uncertainty. *Health Affairs, 3,* 74.

Eddy, D. M. (1992). *A manual for assessing health practices and designing practice policies.* Philadelphia: American College of Physicians.

Horn, S. D. (1995, July). Clinical practice improvement: Improving quality and decreasing cost in managed care. *Medical Interface,* pp. 60–70.

Horn, S. D. (1997). *Clinical practice improvement methodology: Implementation and evaluation.* New York: Faulkner and Gray.

Horn, S. D., Buckle, J. M., & Carver, C. M. (1988). The Ambulatory Severity Index: Development of an ambulatory case mix system. *Journal of Ambulatory Care Management, 11,* 53–62.

Horn, S. D., Sharkey, P. D., Buckle, J. M., Backofen, J. E., Averill, R. F., & Horn, R. A. (1991). The relationship between severity of illness and hospital length of stay and mortality. *Medical Care, 29*, 305–317.

Horn, S. D., Sharkey, P. D., & Gassaway, J. (1996). Managed Care Outcomes Project: Study design, baseline patient characteristics, and outcome measures. *American Journal of Managed Care, 2*(3), 237–247.

Horn, S. D., Sharkey, P. D., & Levy, R. (1995). A managed care pharmacoeconomic research model based on the Managed Care Outcomes Project. *Journal of Pharmacy Practice, 8*(4), 172–177.

Horn, S. D., Sharkey, P. D., Tracy, D. M., Horn, C. E., James, B., & Goodwin, F. (1996). Intended and unintended consequences of HMO cost containment strategies: Results from the Managed Care Outcomes Project. *American Journal of Managed Care, 2*(3), 253–264.

Iezzoni, L. I. (1998). *Risk adjustment for measuring health care outcomes.* Ann Arbor, MI: Health Administration Press.

Kellie, S. E., & Kelly, J. Y. (1991). Medicare peer review organization pre-procedure review criteria. *Journal of the American Medical Association, 265*, 1265–1270.

Kohn, L. T., Corrigan, J. M., & Donaldson, M. S. (Eds.); Committee on Quality of Health Care in America, Institute of Medicine. (2000). *To err is human: Building a safer health system.* Washington, DC: National Academy Press.

Leape, L. L. (2000). Institute of Medicine medical error figures are not exaggerated. *Journal of the American Medical Association, 284*, 95–97.

Leape, L. L., Bates, D. W., Cullen, D. J., Cooper, J., Demonaco, H. J., Gallivan, T., Hallisey, R., Ives, J., Laird, N., Laffel, G., Nemeskal, R., Petersen, L. A., Porter, K., Servi, D., Shea, B. F., Small, S. D., Sweitzer, B. J., Thompson, B. T., & Vander Vliet, M. (1995). Systems analysis of adverse drug events. *Journal of the American Medical Association, 274*, 35–43.

Leape, L. L., Park, R. E., Kahan, J. P., & Brook, R. N. (1992). Group judgments of appropriateness: The effect of panel composition. *Quality Assurance in Health Care, 4*(2), 151–159.

Magi, D., Douglas, J. M., Jr., & Schwartz, J. S. (1996). Doxycycline compared with azithromycin for treating women with genital chlamydia trachomastis infections: An incremental cost-effectiveness analysis. *Annals of Internal Medicine, 124*(4), 389–399.

McDonald, C. J., Weiner, M., & Hui, S. L. (2000). Deaths due to medical errors are exaggerated in Institute of Medicine Report. *Journal of the American Medical Association, 284*, 93–95.

O'Connor, G. T., Plume, S. K., Beck, J. T., Marrin, C.A.S., Nugent, W., & Olmstead, E. M. (1988). What are my chances? It depends on whom you ask: The choice of a prosthetic heart valve. *Journal of Medical Decision Making,* 8(4), 341.

Park, R. E., Fink, A., Brook, R. H., Chassin, M. R., Kahn, K. L., Merrick, N. J., Kosecoff, J., & Solomon, D. H. (1989). Physician ratings of appropriate indications for three procedures: Theoretical indications vs. indications used in practice. *American Journal of Public Health,* 79(4), 445–447.

Perrow, C. (1984). *Normal accidents: Living with high risk technologies.* New York: Basic Books.

Pestotnik, S. L., Classen, D. C., Evans, R. S., & Burke, J. P. (1996). Implementing antibiotic practice guidelines through computer-assisted decision support: Clinical and financial outcomes. *Annals of Internal Medicine,* 124(10), 884–890.

Williamson, J. W., Goldschmidt, P. G., & Jillson, I. A. (1979). *Medical Practice Information Demonstration Project: Final report* (Office of the Secretary of Health, DHEW). Baltimore, MD: Policy Research.

Part Four

Systems Models for Reducing Error

The idea that the causes of both medical error and suboptimal care lie less with the individual clinician and more in the broader organizational system within which the clinician is embedded has taken center stage in the past several years, as is evident in the Institute of Medicine's report *To Err Is Human: Building a Safer Health System*. This sophisticated view has unseated the more traditional view that harm to patients is simply the result of human blunders or, worse, the result of negligence. In part this broader understanding of the causes of errors and failures comes from studies of accidents conducted by disciplines other than medicine: for example, human factors engineering and high reliability organization theory. Researchers in these disciplines have discovered that problems formerly blamed on human fallibility, incompetence, or negligence often can be traced back to preexisting organizational factors (such as team factors, work environment, organizational design, processes and practices, and financial resources and constraints) or institutional factors (such as the economic and regulatory contexts and national health standards), often referred to as *latent conditions*.

Part Four (Chapters Nine, Ten, and Eleven) focuses on the application of models drawn from organization theory and human factors engineering. One theme that runs through the section is that error mitigation arises partly through individual effort and partly because it is enabled by the wider organization in which clinicians function. A second recurring theme is that even though organizational and systems models hold promise for improving patient safety and mitigating errors, they cannot be applied universally. The task for clinicians and managers is to differentiate between situations, to understand the limits of these models, and to tailor them to fit each unique context. Clearly, in spite of intensified public interest in organizational solutions, we need to do more to understand the complexities and idiosyncrasies of health care organizations if we are to effectively apply these models and avoid unintended consequences.

9

The Reduction of Medical Errors Through Mindful Interdependence

Karl E. Weick

The central question that is addressed in this chapter is, why is it so hard to reduce systemic medical errors when they seem to be everywhere? The answer to be proposed is that systemic medical errors are hard to stop because their genesis is hard to spot. And the reason the genesis of these errors is hard to spot is that analysts are using the wrong conceptual tools. The tools in current use drastically underestimate the role of social, organizational, and interpretive conditions in the generation of adverse medical events and in the creation of safer pathways to patient care.

Part of the reason these influential conditions are underestimated is that the literature on medical error is insistent that there is a basic constant in medical care, and that constant is that medical care is administered in systems. For example, the recent Institute of Medicine study titled *To Err Is Human* states that "health care is composed of a large set of interacting systems—paramedic, emergency, ambulatory, inpatient care, and home health care; testing and imaging laboratories; pharmacies; and so forth—that are connected in loosely coupled but intricate networks of individuals, teams, procedures, regulations, communications, equipment and devices that function with diffused management in a variable and uncertain environment" (Kohn, Corrigan, & Donaldson, 2000, p. 137). There are several key ideas here, including multiple systems, loosely coupled networks, interactions among diverse items, diffuse management, and uncertain environments.

All these ideas are certainly relevant to an analysis of medical error. But to sweep all of them under the generic umbrella of *systems* is to compromise understanding in order to drive home the point that the buck stops everywhere in the genesis of medical error. That is a crucial point to make. It is a point made repeatedly throughout this book. The problem is that when this message is embedded in the terminology of systems, the exhortation carries excess baggage that inadvertently shapes analysis. The noun *system* carries the connotation of an entity that is mechanical, orderly, designed, impervious to improvisation, stable, and routinized. What is harder to see when a system vocabulary is employed are dynamic features such as the unfolding of events, variations in the strength and quality of connections (the handing off of a patient from one unit to another, for example), sequences of activities, the ways in which intelligence is woven into work or stripped away from it, the need to reaccomplish routines, and the ways in which problems are sometimes the outcomes of attempted solutions. Even though all these phenomena may be hard to see, they are present when fallible human beings err and compound small oversights into larger adverse events. These dynamic flows of events are influential, whether that influence is articulated or not. To spot these flows and their flaws, observers need to pay attention to *organizing* as well as organizations and *relationships* as well as systems.

The purpose of this chapter is to show why organizing and relationships are so central to error reduction. The first half of the chapter spells out *givens* in relationships, organizations, and error reduction that all organizations, including medical care organizations, have to contend with. It also offers intermittent suggestions about why these givens tend to go unnoticed in medical care organizations. With these givens as context, I then argue that the primary oversight in depictions of medical systems has been the continued neglect of the extent to which mindfulness is present or absent within these systems. This diagnosis is grounded in analyses of comparable organizations where it has been shown that fuller development of processes of mindful attention is associated with greater system safety. As capabilities to deal mindfully with unexpected events increase, people are better able to detect unfolding errors earlier in their development and to contain more fully those errors that do break through defenses. It is concluded that relationships activated heedlessly and attention deployed heedlessly produce a mindless system that often fails to sense developing threats to patient safety. This view of systemic medical errors translates the static, mechanical image of a *medical system* into a more dynamic, human image of *mindful medical interdependence*. This translation of the abstract vocabulary of systems into the more concrete vocabulary of social and organizational interdependence makes the trajectory of medical errors more transparent and the remedies more apparent.

Relational Givens in Medical Interdependence

I opened this chapter with a quotation that presented the idea of medical systems in a cool, somewhat detached tone. Here is another description of those same medical systems that captures more of their heat and relational density: "Medical care is now more intense. With shorter hospital stays, there is rapid turnover of very sick people who require complex investigation and coordination of monitoring and treatment. So often the tragic outcomes which appear in complaints enquiries are caused not by one terrible mistake, but by the cumulative effect of small errors—medical, nursing, organizational and administrative" (Robinson, 1999, p. 254). This description suggests that clinical medicine involves multiple handoffs, with many places where information could fall between the cracks and small errors could go undetected. The description also suggests that from an organizational perspective, practitioners face situations with high production pressure and overload, which makes it likely that they will develop tunnel vision, rigid adherence to routines, reduction in the number of people they consult, regression to overlearned ways of responding, and unanticipated consequences (Staw, Sandelands, & Dutton, 1981).

Linkages between system nodes in the form of handoffs of a patient from one caregiver to another are the relational infrastructure of medical systems. Interactions are fundamental, as is evident in this description: "Safety does not reside in a person, device, or department, but emerges from the interactions of components of a system" (Kohn et al., 2000, p. 49). When interactions occur, they can be more or less mindful, a quality that, as we will see later, plays an important role in whether errors are caught and corrected or allowed to accumulate and enlarge.

An example of a medical system that is sensitive to the importance of handoffs as relational givens is the pediatric intensive care unit at Loma Linda Children's Hospital (LLCH) (adapted from Perkin & van Straelen, 1997). Before 1989, little attention had been given to the transport system that brought patients to LLCH. This despite the fact that almost half of the admissions to this unit were from hospitals that could not treat children to the degree necessary. Interfacility transport of critically ill, potentially unstable children is complex and involves such problems as equipment failure (estimated to be about 2 percent nationally), physiological deterioration to cardiac arrest and death (estimated to occur in about 7 percent of transports), and accidental extubation when the endotracheal tube becomes dislodged. The incidence of consequential events from these sources dropped to zero in the LLCH transport system for the period from 1995 through 1997, a period during which 5,408 patients were transported and only 8 requests for transport were refused. This reduction in consequential events came about through such changes as training attendants to recognize shock in its covert, compensated phase; stabilizing airways at the referring facility before transport was started; using respiratory therapists rather than residents to place the breathing tube in the wind-pipe; and having a physician attending the transport, not so much to perform procedures as to render medical judgments if needed. These changes affected both individual skills and the interdependent activities involved in dealing with unstable patients.

The system implications become even more apparent when you think about what these changes in transport mean for the staff in the intensive care unit itself. Posttransport patients traditionally have about double the mortality rate of those admitted through the emergency department, operating room, or acute care ward. But that's not true at LLCH. When patients enter the critical care unit from the transport unit, they are in better shape than other arrivals. They have less tissue hypoxia when delivered, they spend less time on ventilators, and the time they do spend is at milder ventilator settings. Pediatric intensivists and bedside caregivers inherit fewer complications and errors from transports because of greater mindfulness in the activities and handoffs that occurred before the patient got to them. LLCH has put a human face on its systems, has seen the importance of handoffs done mindfully, and has taken steps to catch errors through closer attention to relational givens.

Organizational Givens in Medical Interdependence

Medical care organizations, such as the Loma Linda Children's Hospital, are in many ways just like any other organization. Although they share many properties with all other organizations, this similarity and its consequences are often overlooked. "Many, if not most physicians in community practice view organizations such as hospitals primarily as platforms for their work and do not see themselves as being part of [the] larger organization" (Kohn et al., 2000, p. 144). Whether overlooked or not, the basics of organizing provide important constraints on error reduction. Barry Turner's summary of the basics of organizing is a credible, economical formulation. He argues that for an organization to be effective, it has to act as a single entity. This requirement for unity is hindered, however, by the diversity of individuals and by the need for internal diversity to cope with external complexities.

To counter this diversity, an organization relies on three mechanisms (Turner, 1978, p. 164):

1. "[I]t establishes a hierarchy of authority and decision-making which enables different problems or subproblems to be considered at different levels of generality within the organization."

2. "[I]t permits those with the greater power in the organization to operate through the formal hierarchy and in other ways to encourage actions, intentions and analyses which they approve of and to discourage conflicting views."

3. "[I]t ensures a continuity of outlook, practice and knowledge within the organization by means of social processes of communication and socialization which enable the organization to build up and maintain a sub-culture embodying the organization's distinctive character and mode of operation."

A person joining an organization accepts "a set of assumptions, criteria, and premises which will serve to guide his decision-making by informing him of the kinds of criteria which are acceptable as rationales for decision-choices within the organization concerned" (p. 165). These premises are intended to give the organization singleness of purpose and integrity of action. These are the very same premises that people have in mind when they talk about a *safety culture* (see, for example, Reason, 1997, chap. 9). These premises contain beliefs about the world and its hazards as well as precautionary norms.

Over time all organizations accumulate unnoticed events that are at odds with their accepted beliefs about hazards and their norms for avoiding those hazards. These unnoticed events are partly encompassed by the well-known concept of latent conditions. *Latent conditions* are events that happen long before accidents, that are removed from the direct control of the frontline operator, and that cause operator errors. Latent conditions include things like poor design, gaps in supervision, incorrect installation, unworkable procedures, shortfalls in training, clumsy automation, poorly structured organizations, faulty maintenance, and bad management decisions (Reason, 1997, p. 10).

All of this is pretty straightforward, just about what you would expect from a designer who tried to create a rational mechanism to coordinate activities. But these rational presumptions are not themselves the givens of organization. Instead, they represent rational intentions that play out much differently when they are actually activated. And it is in the outcomes of behavior intended to be rational where the givens of organizing actually materialize. The difference between intention and outcome can be striking. For example, another way to phrase Turner's point (1978) that organizations enforce a finite set of premises to create unity is to say that "organizations achieve a minimal level of coordination by persuading their decision-makers to agree that they will all neglect the same kinds of consideration when they make decisions" (p. 166). If this *consensual neglect* is taken as a given, then error reduction requires that people pay close attention to these simplifications and oversights to detect possible sources of error.

Although organizations are envisioned as rational designs, in their actual unfolding this rationality takes on a different, more fallible, more human character:

> An alternative perspective [to that of the rational organization] on organizations holds that information is limited and serves largely to justify decisions or positions already taken; goals, preferences and effectiveness criteria are problematic and conflicting; organizations are

loosely linked to their social environments; the rationality of various designs and decisions is inferred after the
fact to make sense out of things that have already happened; organizations are coalitions of various interests;
organization designs are frequently unplanned and are
basically responses to contests among interests for control over the organization; and organization designs are
in part ceremonial. This alternative perspective attempts
explicitly to recognize the social nature of organizations
[Pfeffer & Salancik, 1977, pp. 18–19].

This alternative perspective is not meant to be read as a cyni-
cal indictment of organizations. It is simply an enumeration of the
ways in which fallible people with their own interests organize to
tackle tasks that are beyond their individual capabilities. To improve patient safety is to work with these fallibilities, not deny them.

Notice that as we begin to think more carefully about organizational givens, we begin to see that organizational safety is *not* a
separate issue from organizational production. Both production and
safety depend on the same organizational processes of designing,
constructing, operating, maintaining, selecting, training, supervis-
ing, and managing (Reason, 1997, p. 36). The coexistence of safety
and production is evident in Reason's own treatment of his influential notion of latent conditions. He argues that latent conditions are
present in all systems and are inevitable in organizational life. That
is to be expected because resources are rarely distributed equally
among departments. These "inequities create quality, reliability, or
safety problems for someone somewhere in the system at some later
point" (p. 11). If latent conditions are always present, then there is
a premium on making them visible so that they can be made
correctable.

An additional important given in organizational life is that a
person's position in a structure shapes that person's interpretation

and worldview. People at the top of medical hierarchies see a different world than do those at the bottom. And people at the top often place a high premium on "medical autonomy and perfection and (have) a historical lack of interprofessional cooperation and effective communication" (Kohn et al., 2000, p. 142). These givens of organizational life at the top of medical organizations have effects beyond the obvious ones of difficulty in sharing authority, collaborating in problem solving, and seeing the big picture (p. 155).

The additional effects follow a pattern. The higher in a hierarchy an error occurs and the more orderly the organization, the more likely it is that the error will be magnified, the more likely it is that the error will be compounded with other errors, and the more likely it is that the error will be disastrous. Turner (1978) describes a similar idea this way: "Those errors which arise at higher levels within an organization are likely both to be more far-reaching, and to be associated with more complex kinds of accidents. They are likely to be more far-reaching because the higher an error is when it occurs, the more likely it is to be disseminated through the amplifying power of the organization; they are likely to be more complex because higher-level errors are more likely to pick up and combine with smaller, lower-level errors that, by themselves, would not have produced anything untoward" (p. 187). Reason (1997) has made a similar argument. He asserts that operators inherit system defects laid down earlier and higher by acts and decisions involving issues such as resource allocation, inadequate training, scheduling, spatial coordination, and feedback.

A good example of what happens when the givens of organization are ignored is found in Ron Westrum's analysis (1982) of the continuing problems pediatricians had in "seeing" child abuse. Pediatricians are near the top of medical hierarchies. Early suspicions that parents might be injuring their children were voiced by radiologists, people potentially lower in the hierarchy. These radiologists saw multiple fractures at different stages of healing in children, yet parents had no memory of what had happened. These findings were rarely discussed with pediatricians. And when they were, pediatricians were skeptical of the idea that parents were battering their children. Instead, pediatricians continued to make diagnoses such as "brittle bones," "bruises easily," and "subject to spontaneous brain bleeds." Pediatricians essentially said to themselves, "If parents were battering their children, I would know about it. And because I don't know about it, it isn't happening." Westrum calls this the *fallacy of centrality*. It is the belief that one is at the center of an information network rather than just one interdependent player among many in a complex system. The reality is that systems have lots of centers, each with its own unique expertise, simplifications, and blind spots. It is the exchanging and coordinating of the information distributed among these centers that separates more from less intelligent systems. Systems that fail to coordinate effectively, and systems in which people assume that things they don't know about are not material, tend toward higher error rates.

As a footnote to the child abuse example, it is interesting that the pieces of the battered child puzzle were not put together until social workers (people low in the medical hierarchy) were added to the pediatric treatment teams at the University of Colorado. Pediatricians and radiologists were uncertain what they should do next if they did see parental abuse, so they were reluctant to see it. Social workers, however, did know how to engage protective services and how to deal with abusive parents. Once their capability was added to the treatment team, physicians could afford to see battered children because now they could do something about them.

There is an important lesson here for error reduction. People tend to see what they are able to deal with. If a team enlarges what it can do, then it may also enlarge what it will see. A team that sees more has a better chance to see small errors earlier and to do something about them. Small improvements in seeing can occur when individuals enlarge their personal repertoires of what they can do.

But larger improvements in seeing should occur when people with more diverse skills, experience, and perspectives think together in a context of respectful interaction. Again, we see the central importance of organizing for greater mindfulness in medical care.

Error Reduction Givens in Medical Interdependence

In the earlier discussion of latent conditions, I used an innocent-appearing phrase that points to a central given in error reduction. I said that latent events such as unworkable procedures materialize long before accidents and "cause operator errors." The direction of causality is what is crucial here. Human error is a consequence of flawed organizing rather than a major cause of accidents (Reason, 1997, p. 126). This is a central point in organizational analyses. Postmortems of medical errors tend to focus too much on the last few minutes and the last error just before the adverse event, and too little on the contributions to error that were laid down in the preceding days and decisions and that made these last few minutes so harrowing and inevitable.

But the fact that human errors are a consequence rather than a cause of adverse events is not the only given in error reduction. Equally basic is the fact that humans are not perfect. As Reason (1997, p. 25) says in discussing aviation, "human fallibility is like gravity, weather, and terrain, just another foreseeable hazard." The pervasiveness of error would not even be worth mentioning were it not for the fact that medicine is often driven by the idea that perfection is possible and that mistakes are a personal and professional failure. This perfection mind-set, just like the mind-set that tries to design a rational organization, is laudable, admirable, and unworkable. Both mind-sets produce glaring blind spots. People imbued with the idea of perfection are unable to see that errors are normal, that errors are opportunities to learn, and that human beings have strengths as well as limitations. *To Err Is Human* notes, for example, that "human beings have many intellectual strengths, such as their large memory capacity; a large repertory of responses; flexibility in applying these responses to information inputs; and an ability to react creatively and effectively to the unexpected. However, human beings also have well-known limitations, including difficulty in attending carefully to several things at once, difficulty in recalling detailed information quickly, and generally poor computational ability" (Kohn et al., 2000, p. 146). Later, I show how organizing for mindfulness counteracts limitations such as these. For the moment, the point is simply that people are prone to make errors. And the kinds of errors they make on routine tasks are different from those they make on nonroutine tasks (p. 140).

Given an organization of fallible human beings, the issue is *not* why does an error occur, but rather, why wasn't the error corrected. "A reliable system has procedures and attributes that make errors visible to those working in the system so that they can be corrected before causing harm" (Kohn et al., 2000, p. 152). There are at least two issues here, error visibility and error correction. And neither one is straightforward because a lot is at stake. Diane Vaughan (1996) found how high these stakes were when she took a close look at the *Challenger* disaster: "When an unexpected event occurs, we need to explain it not only to others, but to ourselves. So we imbue it with meaning in order to make sense of it. We correct history, reconstructing the past so that it will be consistent with the present, reaffirming our sense of self and place in the world. We reconstruct history every day, not to fool others but to fool ourselves, because it is integral to the process of going on. People attempt to rescue order from disorder" (p. 281). When an unexpected event occurs, we first have to notice it, then we have to make sense of it, and finally we have to do something about it. Adverse medical events materialize due to failures in each of these processes. And remedies lie in heightened mindfulness at the transitions between each of these steps.

People can't remedy problems that they don't know exist. And there is reasonable evidence that medical personnel fall short in noticing errors, in making sense of them as events to be taken seriously, and in enacting remedies. Medical personnel are often confused about what constitutes an error and what should be reported, even when fear of reprisal is low (Augustine, Weick, Bagian, & Lee, 1998). Surgical morbidity and mortality (M and M) reviews are conducted with highly variable thoroughness, are seen as important and powerful educational tools by less than half of those in attendance (43 percent of residents and 47 percent of surgical faculty), are given even lower rankings for their "value in reducing error and improving care," and "tend not to address systemic issues" (Kohn et al., 2000, p. 220). The picture is one of halfhearted inquiry that is unlikely to spot errors and even less likely to spot remedies. The same goes for the 40 percent discrepancy between antemortem and postmortem diagnoses and the reluctance to use these data to improve noticing, sensemaking, or action (p. 221). But even when problems are noticed, such as the disturbingly high yet stable (p. 220) incidence of nosocomial infections (infections acquired while in health care that are unrelated to the original condition), remedial actions such as handwashing occur with modest frequency. Medical care that is mindful of patient safety through the practice of handwashing is not much further along than it was at the time Semmelweis first urged handwashing to reduce mortality at childbirth, and first encountered system barriers to implementation (Nuland, 1979).

The failure to use settings devoted to medical inquiry as a robust forum to create safer patient care is an even bigger lost opportunity than medical personnel may realize. The lost opportunity arises from a subtle peculiarity in the design of safe operating procedures. When people focus on procedures themselves, then the steps necessary to produce efficient work tend to arise fairly naturally from the combination of the equipment, the task, and the goals. This configuration tends to prompt the person about what should be done next and encourages a flow of action. But this combination of naturalness and inevitability that leads into the next step in efficient work disappears when the issue shifts to the design of *safe* work. Safe procedures tend to be defined in terms of *actions prohibited*. The danger then is that when people pursue safe work, the range of permitted actions will shrink until it is smaller than the range necessary to get the job done (Reason, 1997, p. 49). When this shrinkage occurs, people are forced to take shortcuts and violate prohibitions. And when they take shortcuts, they are just as likely to omit central steps in procedures as peripheral ones. Thus an intention to create safer practice through prohibition may in fact make that practice more dangerous than it was before. Experts are in a good position to stop this dangerous spiral. They often see means other than simple prohibition as pathways to safer practice. Thus, when M and M reviews are perfunctory, organizations lose a chance to improve patient safety through process redesign rather than prohibition.

Two final givens in error reduction underscore how crucial awareness is for patient safety and how dangerous the uneven distribution of awareness is. First, safety is a dynamic nonevent (Weick, 1987). When things are going right, nothing adverse is happening. The huge trap here is the inference that because nothing adverse is happening, nothing is being done to create this nonoccurrence. That inference is wrong. The continuing absence of adverse events is the result of continuing adjustments to ongoing variations, any one of which, if ignored, could escalate into a serious problem. Chronic wariness is the tone in a safe system. Hubris is the enemy.

Second, neither safety nor reliability is bankable. "Unless continual reinvestments are made in improving technical systems, procedures, reporting processes, and employee attentiveness, those performance standards that have already been attained are likely to degrade" (Schulman, 1993, p. 35). Again we see how closely safety is intertwined with production. Good management that creates effective organizations is indistinguishable from mindful management that creates safe organizations.

Toward Mindful Error Correction
in Medical Care

Throughout the preceding discussion, there are scattered references to mindfulness, awareness, and alertness as scarce organizational resources that are indispensable to increased patient safety. This final section pulls these scattered references together into a coherent conceptual scheme that makes it easier for people to see an organizational infrastructure for error reduction.

The central concept to be discussed is *mindfulness*. By mindfulness, I mean a rich awareness of discriminatory detail. This rich awareness is a mixture of active differentiation and refinement of existing distinctions; creation of new, discontinuous categories out of the continuous flow of activity; and a deep, nuanced appreciation of the context and of alternative ways to deal with it (adapted from Langer, 1989). It is the contention of this chapter that mindfulness arises from two sources: care in interrelating and care in directing attention to the unexpected. People may carry out interrelating heedfully yet be distracted from giving close attention to the unexpected because they are already giving close attention to production pressures. Likewise, they may focus on discriminatory detail with heedful attentiveness yet fail to extrapolate that detail to potential consequences for the system and also fail to embed that detail in altered contributions and representations. However, disconnects such as these are uncommon when there is highly effective organizing for high reliability. What is more common, as I discuss later, is that reliable performance reduces error. And this error reduction is the outcome of ongoing mindfulness, which itself is a product of heedful interrelating and heedful attentiveness.

Thus the central idea that derives from unpacking the *system* metaphor is that effective error reduction in medical care is more likely when relationships embody ongoing mindfulness. This conclusion is based on investigations of organizations such as nuclear-powered aircraft carriers, nuclear power plants, financial institutions, chemical manufacturers, and air traffic control, all of whom share with medicine a potential for adverse events that materialize from unexpected accumulations of uncorrected errors. Medicine is not unique among these industries, because it too is concerned with "learning how to prevent, detect, recover, and learn from accidents" (Kohn et al., 2000, p. 137). And these industry leaders have shown an unusual ability to understand hazardous conditions and to reduce vulnerability based on this understanding.

Among these leading organizations, the one that furnishes the analogy for this section is the same one that was singled out by the Institute of Medicine (Kohn et al., 2000, pp. 138–139) for its unique relevance to medical organizations, namely, aircraft carriers (for example, Weick & Roberts, 1993). The circumstances surrounding flight operations on the decks of aircraft carriers bear a close resemblance to the health care environment. In both settings there are risks created when incompatible activities must be performed in close proximity (for example, aircraft are fueled and loaded with bombs while their engines are running and the deck is pitching in the waves). There are also the similarities of the "huge variability in patients and circumstances, the need to adapt processes quickly, the quickly changing knowledge base, and the importance of highly trained professional who must use expert judgment in dynamic settings" (Kohn et al., 2000, p. 138). Initial analyses of aircraft carriers (for example, Rochlin, LaPorte, & Roberts, 1987) suggested that carrier personnel were able to avoid serious injury and the destruction of aircraft because they gave top priority to safety, designed redundancy into the system, implemented a safety culture, trained personnel continuously, and emphasized learning from those incidents that did happen (Kohn et al., 2000, p. 49). These findings, which are the centerpiece of *high reliability theory*, represent an overview of important targets in safety improvement.

When my colleagues and I took a closer look at these highly reliable organizations (Weick & Roberts, 1993; Weick, Sutcliffe, & Obstfeld, 1999; Weick & Sutcliffe, 2001), we saw something that had been missed in earlier analyses. We saw that there was a distinctive character to the way in which people related among themselves and to their work. When they interrelated their separate activities, they did so heedfully, taking special care to enact their actions as *contributions* to a system rather than as simply tasks in their autonomous individual jobs. Their heedful interrelating also was reflected in the care they directed toward accurate *representation* of the other players and their contributions. And heedful interrelating was evident in the care they directed toward *subordinating* their idiosyncratic intentions to the effective functioning of the system (what was good for the system was good for them). When interrelating was done heedfully, there was an increase in the alertness and intelligence that was mobilized to deal with the unexpected. And errors decreased. The resulting *mind* of this system, the emergent capability to get on top of the unexpected more quickly, did not lie inside the head of any one person. Instead, the mind was located between people, in the quality of their relating.

Although all of this may sound a bit far-fetched, that is mostly because it is tough to envision and describe the social character of systems, especially if one is prone to see the world as a place of individual heroics and tangible machinery. Yet as I discussed earlier, it is that very social character of systems, that very fact that ties are enacted heedfully or heedlessly, that determines whether errors are corrected or passed along. The dynamics described here as characteristic of high-performing crews on carrier decks are not that different from the dynamics of a high-performing medical team: "People make fewer errors when they work in teams. When processes are planned and standardized, each member knows his or her responsibilities as well as those of teammates, and members 'look out' for one another noticing errors before they cause an accident" (Kohn et al., 2000, p. 150). One can talk about contributions or one can talk about people's knowing their team responsibilities, one can talk about representation or about people's knowing the responsibilities of their teammates, and one can talk about subordination or about team members' looking out for one another and for harbingers of accidents. The analyses are equivalent, as are the implicit requirements for safer practice.

So far I have described a recurrent way in which relationships seemed to be structured in high reliability organizations, labeling this recurrence *heedful interrelating*. What was striking about this structuring was that it functioned as if it were a mind. Intelligence was added to operations by the care with which people coordinated their activities and remained attentive to the quality of that coordinating. They acted in ways that suggested they were mindful of the relational givens mentioned earlier. Their actions also suggested a tacit understanding that these ways of interrelating had to be accomplished over and over again, because they tended to unravel. And people also seemed to understand that relations are especially prone to unraveling when those doing the interrelating prize individuality and autonomy.

But what is still missing from this emerging picture of collective mind is content. There is heedful connecting, but of what? Heedful interrelating creates mindfulness, but that mindfulness must exist as more than a general capability. To focus that mindfulness on issues of safety and reliability requires an additional set of processes. What is interesting about these additional processes, at least the ones found in high reliability organizations, is that they too generate mindfulness. Thus, high reliability organizations are distinguished by the fact that they are mindful twice over. Both how they act (heedful interrelating) and what they do (heedful attending) reflect a commitment to mindful performance. It is conceivable that it is this high degree of mindfulness, as much as the explicit preoccupation with safety, that explains the dramatic success that high reliability systems have in managing errors.

Heedful attending is embodied in five processes that show up repeatedly in organizations that successfully contain errors. High reliability systems are heedfully attentive to failures, simplifications, operations, resilience, and distributed expertise. These five are especially noteworthy in the context of medical errors, because they represent specific practices that can be initiated immediately in order to gain indirect leverage on error correction through direct leverage on alertness. The following five processes can be thought of as hard-won lessons in the continuing *struggle for alertness* that high reliability organizations face every day. They are the constants that enable organizations to manage variations they never anticipated.

1. *Preoccupation with failure.* Systems with higher reliability worry chronically that analytical errors are embedded in ongoing activities and that unexpected failure modes and limitations of foresight may amplify those analytical errors. The people who operate and manage high reliability organizations "assume that each day will be a bad day and act accordingly. But this is not an easy state to sustain, particularly when the thing about which one is uneasy has either not happened, or has happened a long time ago, and perhaps to another organization" (Reason, 1997, p. 37). These systems have been characterized as consisting of "collective bonds among suspicious individuals." They have also been described as places that institutionalize disappointment (Landau & Chisholm, 1995). To institutionalize disappointment means, in the words of the head of pediatric critical care at Loma Linda Children's Hospital, "to constantly entertain the thought that we have missed something" (Perkin & van Straelen, 1997).

2. *Reluctance to simplify interpretations.* All organizations have to ignore most of what they see in order to get work done. The crucial issue is whether their simplified diagnoses force them to ignore key sources of unexpected difficulties. Mindful of the importance of this trade-off, systems with higher reliability restrain their temptations to simplify. They do so through such means as diverse checks and balances, adversarial reviews, intentional creation of learning contexts (Edmondson, 1996), and cultivation of multiple perspectives. At the Diablo Canyon nuclear power plant, for example, people preserve complexity in their interpretations and head off

simplification by reminding themselves of two things: (a) we have not yet experienced all potential failure modes that could occur here, and (b) we have not yet deduced all potential failure modes that could occur here (Schulman, 1993). These people know that their enemy is hubris. And they know that optimism is the height of arrogance.

3. *Sensitivity to operations*. People in systems with higher reliability tend to pay close attention to operations. Everyone, no matter what his or her level, values organizing in order to maintain situational awareness. Resources are deployed so that people can see what is happening, can comprehend what it means, and can project into the near future what these understandings predict will happen. In medical care settings, sensitivity to operations often means that the system is organized to support the bedside caregiver.

4. *Cultivation of resilience*. Most systems try to anticipate trouble spots, but the higher reliability systems also pay close attention to their capability to investigate, learn, and act without knowing in advance what people will be called to act on (adapted from Wildavsky, 1991, p. 70). Reliable systems spend time improving their capacity to do a quick study, to develop swift trust, to engage in just-in-time learning, to simulate mentally, and to work with fragments of potentially relevant past experience. Resilience and skilled improvisation tend to go hand in hand.

5. *Willingness to organize around expertise*. One of the more striking properties of reliable systems is their willingness to let decisions *migrate* to those with the expertise to make them. Adherence to rigid hierarchies is loosened, especially during high-tempo periods, so that there is a better matching of experience with problems. For example, at Loma Linda Children's Hospital the problem of accidental extubations of the endotracheal tube is handled as follows. "When the nurse believes that the child's agitation may cause tube dislodgment she asks the resident for an order to increase sedation and/or paralysis. Residents have been taught to respect the nurses'

recommendations. Requests by the nurse for an increase in medication are not denied" (Perkin & van Straelen, 1997, p. 3).

Conclusion

What can medical people do right now to begin to reduce medical errors?

The best answer I have heard comes from Winston Churchill. During World War II Churchill made a colossal error when he failed to realize how vulnerable Singapore was to attack by a Japanese land invasion. This error led to Singapore's downfall. In Churchill's equivalent of an M and M review after Singapore's collapse, he asked four questions, every one of them a systems question. He asked: why didn't I know? why wasn't I told? why didn't I ask? why didn't I tell what I knew? (Allinson, 1993, pp. 11–12). Those four questions are questions of interdependence. They take seriously the idea that knowledge is not something people possess in their heads but rather something people do together. And as this chapter has discussed, an important source of medical errors seems to be the extreme variation with which people enact mindful interdependencies.

There is no substitute for greater sensitivity to the ways in which medical activities are interrelated. Those relationships, those handoffs, are where errors accumulate or are caught. Those are the moments that can make or break a profession. The good news in this line of thinking is that there are leverage points in medical systems where error reduction is possible. The bad news is that those leverage points are not where people think they are. What is laudable among medical professionals is their tendency to attack the problem of medical errors by working to improve their individual technical skills. But the locus of the problem lies upstream and downstream from the skilled individual. It lies in the organizing and the connecting of activities. Adverse events build up along the contours of interdependence. If that interdependence is flawed, then brilliant individuals may be rendered incompetent. Shortfalls in either heedful interrelating or heedful attentiveness lead to heightened vulnerability, slower error correction, and the development of more serious problems.

Considering medical errors in this light is to gain at least two conceptual advantages. First, this way of posing the issue of medical errors is consistent with the givens of relations, organizations, and errors. Second, this way of posing the issue of medical errors avoids the undifferentiated image of systems and preserves the reality of pervasive interdependence in medical care. This substitution of heedful processes for generic systems makes for richer description. And the substitution of collective mindfulness for individual mindfulness makes for fuller detection. Both of these substitutions can pave the way to a more confident and pragmatic line of action that produces greater patient safety.

That's the message from organizational studies.

References

Allinson, R. E. (1993). *Global disasters*. Upper Saddle River, NJ: Prentice Hall.

Augustine, C. H., Weick, K. E., Bagian, J. P., & Lee, C. Z. (1998, November). Predispositions toward a culture of safety in a large multi-facility health system. Paper presented at the Annenberg Center for Health Sciences conference *Enhancing Patient Safety and Reducing Errors in Health Care*, Rancho El Mirage, CA.

Edmondson, A. C. (1996). Learning from mistakes is easier said than done: Group and organizational influences on the detection and correction of human error. *Journal of Applied Behavioral Science, 32*(1), 5–28.

Kohn, L. T., Corrigan, J. M., & Donaldson, M. S. (Eds.); Committee on Quality of Health Care in America, Institute of Medicine. (2000). *To err is human: Building a safer health system*. Washington, DC: National Academy Press.

Landau, M., & Chisholm, D. (1995). The arrogance of optimism: Notes on failure avoidance management. *Journal of Contingencies and Crisis Management, 3*, 67–80.

Langer, E. (1989). Minding matters: The consequences of mindlessness-mindfulness. In L. Berkowitz (Ed.), *Advances in experimental social psychology* (Vol. 22, pp. 137–173). New York: Academic Press.

Nuland, S. B. (1979). The enigma of Semmelweis: An interpretation. *Journal of the History of Medicine, 34*(3), 255–272.

Perkin, R. M., & van Straelen, D. (1997). *Pediatric critical care in Loma Linda Children's Hospital.* Unpublished manuscript.

Pfeffer, J., & Salancik, G. R. (1977, Autumn). Organizational design: The case for a coalition model of organizations. *Organizational Dynamics, 6,* 15.

Reason, J. (1997). *Managing the risks of organizational accidents.* Aldershot, UK: Ashgate.

Robinson, J. (1999). The price of deceit: The reflections of an advocate. In M. M. Rosenthal, L. Mulcahy, & S. Lloyd-Bostock (Eds.), *Medical mishaps: Pieces of the puzzle* (pp. 246–256). Bristol, PA: Open University Press.

Rochlin, G., LaPorte, T., & Roberts, K. (1987). The self-designing high reliability organization: Aircraft carrier flight operation at sea. *Naval War College Review, 40,* 76–90.

Schulman, P. R. (1993). The analysis of high reliability organizations: A comparative framework. In K. H. Roberts (Ed.), *New challenges to understanding organizations* (pp. 33–53). New York: Macmillan.

Staw, B. M., Sandelands, L. E., & Dutton, J. E. (1981). Threat-rigidity effects in organizational behavior: A multi-level analysis. *Administrative Science Quarterly, 26,* 501–524.

Turner, B. (1978). *Man-made disasters.* London: Wykeham.

Vaughan, D. (1996). *The Challenger launch decision.* Chicago: University of Chicago Press.

Weick, K. E. (1987). Organizational culture as a source of high reliability. *California Management Review, 29,* 112–127.

Weick, K. E., & Roberts, K. H. (1993). Collective mind in organizations: Heedful interrelating on flight decks. *Administrative Science Quarterly, 38,* 357–381.

Weick, K. E., & Sutcliffe, K. M. (2001). *Managing the unexpected: Assuring high performance in an age of complexity.* San Francisco: Jossey-Bass.

Weick, K. E., Sutcliffe, K. M., & Obstfeld, D. (1999). Organizing for high reliability: Processes of collective mindfulness. In B. Staw & R. Sutton (Eds.), *Research in organizational behavior* (Vol. 21, pp. 81–123). Greenwich, CT: JAI.

Westrum, R. (1982). Social intelligence about hidden events. *Knowledge, 3*(3), 381–400.

Wildavsky, A. (1991). *Searching for safety.* New Brunswick, NJ: Transaction.

10

Medical Errors
How Reliable Is Reliability Theory?

Paul R. Schulman

The release of *To Err Is Human* (Kohn, Corrigan, & Donaldson, 2000), the Institute of Medicine (IOM) report on medical errors, and the resulting public pronouncements, policy proposals, and reactions from health care organizations pose both an opportunity and a dilemma. The opportunity is to highlight an important problem in the U.S. health care system, bring new information to bear on it, and as we all hope, gain some improvement. The dilemma is that medical error is a problem that confronts directly the limits of our knowledge about human reliability in organized settings.

What does organization theory have to contribute to our understanding of medical errors? In its report to the president, based on the findings of the IOM study, the federal Quality Interagency Coordination Task Force (2000) asserts that "the majority of medical errors today are not produced by negligence, lack of education, or lack of training. Rather, errors occur in our health care systems due to poor systems design and organizational factors, much as in any other industry" (p. 36). Organization theory, particularly that devoted to reliability, suggests that this assertion itself might constitute something of a medical error—it confuses as much as it clarifies.

Recognizing a Reliability Spectrum: Marginal Reliability Versus the Reliability of Precluded Events

Organizations can adopt a variety of approaches and strategies for promoting reliability in their internal processes (Rochlin & Von Meier, 1994; Schulman, 1993a; Weick, Sutcliffe, & Obstfeld, 1999; Wildavsky, 1988). If there is a generalization that emerges from the growing number of reliability analyses it would seem to be this: successful organizational approaches to reliability are determined both by the properties of the failures an organization seeks to avoid and by the stability of the environmental equilibrium the organization has achieved with respect to those failures. These issues in the context of medical error are the subjects of this chapter.

We know that every pattern of organization is only a partial "solution" to the purposes or goals of organizing. In any organizational design some values are organized in, but other values just as surely are organized out. The same is true of reliability. If we organize to be more reliable this must come at some cost to another value — speed, output, or possibly efficiency. The same is true of the types of errors we attempt to be reliable about. We can try to organize to prevent *errors of omission*—errors in which no action or delayed action is taken when fast action is required. This is usually accomplished by procedures that mandate action, punishment for inaction, and perhaps even organizational reinforcement of heroic actions taken by individuals (Schulman, 1996). But organizing to protect against errors of omission increases the likelihood of *errors of commission*— acting too soon, before all the facts are in.[1] An organization cannot protect against one type of error without making its reciprocal error more likely.

Broadly speaking, strategies for the promotion of reliability in organizations can be arrayed along a continuum bounded by two extremes. On the one hand we can identify a strategy of *marginal reliability*, a strategy in which reliability is traded off at the margins in exchange for other dominant organizational values such as efficiency, productivity, and the like. In this case, the organization promotes reliability probabilistically—measures are taken to reduce the trend of errors over a large number of repetitive processes, yet it is recognized that in any particular case error is still possible.

On the other hand an organization can attempt to identify those events (such as a reactor core meltdown or a midair collision of two commercial aircraft under air traffic control) that simply must not happen at any frequency. These are events whose occurrence would threaten not only large numbers of lives but the stability or survival of the organization itself. These are events the members of an organization wish not simply to elude probabilistically but to preclude deterministically. We can label this approach to reliability the *reliability of precluded events*.

Recent research in the reliability of organizations has focused on this latter reliability challenge (LaPorte & Consolini, 1991; Roberts, 1993; Sanne, 2000; Schulman, 1993b). The thrust of this work has been the identification and analysis of a set of high-performance organizations that must maintain high levels of operational reliability and safety in the management of very hazardous systems, systems about which there is a great deal of public dread. For each of these organizations, the pursuit of high levels of day-to-day reliability and safety is a requirement for survival in the unforgiving political and regulatory niche it occupies.

But most organizations can be successful by addressing marginal reliability. For these organizations the reliability of key activities and processes, including the likelihood of accidents and injuries, is understood and valued within the context of overall production output and efficiency. Accidents and errors either reduce or destroy output or increase overall costs associated with producing a given product. Accidents and failures thus affect the balance between costs and output. Reliability conceived in this way can be adjusted at the margins—the marginal costs of reliability or safety improvements can be weighed against their impact on the likelihood of increased production.

To be sure, the imposition of liability and regulatory standards means that a pure efficiency standard cannot be applied, but insurance and the payment of regulatory fines can be factored into efficiency calculations. The reliability traded off on behalf of other values is accepted as part of a more or less stable equilibrium between the organization and the societal environment in which it operates.

Another factor that makes a marginal reliability strategy possible is that marginal shifts in the commitment of resources can be closely grounded in a mass of accumulated organizational experience. Lots of errors, production lapses, and accidents over time build a base of experiential knowledge from which the organization can determine the resource commitments likely to yield some marginal improvement. Whether these changes are worth their costs is the key reliability decision.

Now, at the other end of the reliability spectrum are organizations in sharply different circumstances. These are the organizations that face technical hazards in their operations that render certain events literally unendurable. Either the organization and its assets would be destroyed by the event, or social and political reaction would force a major transformation of the organization if not its termination. Again, these are events such as a nuclear weapons accident, a reactor core meltdown, or a major midair collision of commercial jets under air traffic control. The public dread of these accidents is so great that even *precursor events*, which suggest their possibility, are likely to have threatening consequences.[2]

These latter organizations occupy highly precarious social, political, and legal niches, survival in which may well demand that given events simply not happen. Under these circumstances, reliability assessments are quite different from those connected to production efficiency, in fact they are often detached from issues of output altogether. Generally these organizations are shielded from market pressures that would impose the trading off of values such as efficiency with reliability. They are often governmental organizations, as in the case of air traffic control centers and nuclear weapons agencies, or they are buffered from full market competition by regulation or subsidies or both, as in the case of nuclear power or commercial aviation companies.

For an organization confronted by reliability challenges of this order, reliability becomes in effect a nonmarginalizable organizational property. Few explicit efficiency trade-offs, even marginal ones, surrounding precluded events are acceptable to key players in the organization's environment. Perhaps a nuclear power plant could get along with one less redundant diesel generator for emergency reactor shutdown, but such plants must ask how this option will sit with regulators, antinuclear groups, and an anxious public.

In addition, organizations committed to reliability against precluded events do not have the knowledge base that would support fine-grained reliability trade-offs at the margins. Precluded events very rarely happen. A variety of precursor events do occur, of course, and these do increase knowledge, but their linkage to the most critical failures and precluded events is idiosyncratic and uncertain. Trial-and-error learning about these linkages is not a practical possibility. The first error is likely to be the last trial (LaPorte, 1996).

In the statistical modeling of complex causal relationships, the validity of findings depends in the first instance on having an appropriate balance between variables and cases. If there are many variables to assess and only a few data points, the model is *overdetermined* and the independent contribution of any variable to the cases is hard to establish. This comes close to describing the information base of organizations committed to the reliability of precluded events. They are complex technical and organizational systems, with many variables in play. Yet they have, and must have, a very small number of cases of significant failure—few data points—over which to sort out which variable contributes to what. To be sure, much information is gathered about precluded events by hypothetical means—simulations, fault-tree analysis, probabilistic risk assessment, and the like. But these efforts do not produce a deep enough picture of operations to connect a specific change with an observable effect—especially when the effect is only a shift in the probability of a nonevent.

What reliability becomes for an organization that escalates it to the level of precluded events is a *holistic* property. Reliability may thus be treated as if it were a variable whose proxy is overall organizational health. Because members of the organization cannot pinpoint causation, cannot differentiate and bound a limited set of reliability or safety variables, they must see everything as a potential factor in a dangerous incident, either as a triggering element or a root cause.[3] This means that the commitment to reliability for such an organization may not be subject to clear end points or *stopping rules*. A consistent tending toward organizational well orderedness is the clearest way for managers to assure themselves that they are doing their best to ward off complex causal chains of error or failure that could lead to catastrophic conclusions.

The reliability of precluded events has another unusual property. It is a *prospective* reliability that is not retrospectively established by a good performance record. The past avoidance of precluded events does not constitute an organizational asset of goodwill or credibility that can be banked against future contingencies. These organizations, in their environmental niches, are only as reliable as the first catastrophe that lies ahead of them, not the years of successful operations that may lie behind.

Table 10.1 summarizes the differences between the two ends of the organizational reliability spectrum.

Table 10.1. Marginal Reliability Versus the Reliability of Precluded Events.

Marginal Reliability	Precluded Event Reliability
Context of efficiency	Context of social dread
Concentrated risk	Widely distributed risk
Marginal calculation	Holistic analysis
Stable trade-offs	No formal stopping rules
Trial-and-error learning	Logic, analogical learning
Retrospectively determined	Prospectively determined
Probabilistic control	Deterministic control

The Special Case of Medical Errors

It should be evident from this analysis that neither end of the re-liability spectrum effectively describes the case of medical errors. When the IOM report asserts that most medical errors are "systems related," it means they are not attributable to individual negligence or misconduct. But the reliability of precluded events is a strategy directed toward errors with both system-level causes *and large-scale organizational and societal consequences*.

Some medical errors (such as those that could spread dangerous infections widely throughout a hospital and into a surrounding community or those in the handling of nuclear materials) might approach these system-level consequences. But the errors of concern in the IOM report and to medical personnel, regulators, and policy-makers are those centering around the individual patient. Although these errors, even those leading to the death of a patient, certainly intensely affect family members, both psychologically and eco-nomically, they are not system-level errors of the kind rooted in the social dread that demands precluding events. The individual patient at the center of medical error both dramatizes the error and simul-taneously bounds it. Medical procedures may be tightly coupled, with one action or effect leading closely to another (Perrow, 1984), but the first-order effects of medical error generally do not extend far beyond the individual patient.

It seems clear further that no medical organization has in the past or is likely in the immediate future to attempt the deterministic approach of specifying a set of errors that must be avoided independent of costs. The very calculation of recovery rates, death rates, and the like for given medical procedures indicates that adverse medical events (which include errors) are indeed tolerated, both by medical organizations and, more important, by their patients and society.

There are other important differences between medical processes and the processes of deterministic reliability strategies. For one thing, social pressures for medical "production" in the face of risk are far different from those for production by, say, nuclear power or air traffic control organizations. The dread of error in these latter areas far exceeds the demand for production. It is unacceptable to say, for example, "Damn the risks, we need the electric power," or, "Whatever the risks, we need to get this flight in the air." It is perfectly acceptable, and in fact mandated by regulatory agencies, for organizations employing a precluded event reliability strategy to stop output or production in the face of risk. The bias here, both organizational and societal, is in the direction of inaction and the shutting down of systems as opposed to operating them in unsafe conditions. Nuclear power plants *scram*, or shut down a reactor, when conditions escalate risk. Air traffic controllers refuse clearances for planes to take off or keep planes out of a sector when congestion or equipment failures increase risk.

But the demand for medical services is not similarly elastic with respect to safety conditions. When people really need medical attention, they rarely wish to forego it out of concern for the risk of error. It is very rare for a hospital, particularly one that is the only service provider, to have the option of a safety stand-down in the face of error or risk. For individual medical practitioners, errors of intervention are far preferable to errors of omission, and the bias in medical organizations is in the direction of intervention and action.

An additional difference between medical organizations and organizations that pursue the highest reliability approach lies in the predictability of their core technologies. A foundation of high reliability in the latter is the standardization of processes and parts and the existence of a knowledge base that makes the mechanical systems under control highly predictable. In contrast, the raw material for the medical production process is essentially idiosyncratic. The conditions under which services are provided can vary significantly, from emergency to routine. Our knowledge base covering living systems does not provide the degree of predictability we have found for mechanical systems. A number of medical errors are likely to be *forced errors*—errors made under the pressure of having to apply medical processes under crisis conditions of incomplete information, time pressure, and unpredictable patient behavior.

Finally, for organizations committed to the reliability of precluded events, the overwhelming hazards inherent in certain technical systems have produced wide agreement on the definition and identification of *error*. For medical organizations, however, the situation is quite different. For example, in its report *Doing What Counts for Patient Safety: Federal Actions to Reduce Medical Errors and Their Impact*, the Quality Interagency Coordination Task Force (2000) admitted that "the absence of standardized definitions of medical error . . . and the difficulty in distinguishing preventable errors from currently unavoidable adverse events hamper our understanding of this problem" (p. 37). In a revealing sociological study of errors among surgeons in a large Western hospital, Charles Bosk (1979) noted that "error is an 'essentially contested' concept. By this I mean the grounds for fixing the label 'error' to any action are always arguable. In two similar cases with identical outcomes one person may be considered guilty of an error while the other is blameless" (p. 28).

Yet despite all these differences between the circumstances of medical organizations and organizations that practice the reliability of precluded events, medical errors are not fully marginalizable either. Major medical practitioners subscribe to an oath to help others and *to do no harm*. In the environment of medical organizations, malpractice suits and medical scandals intensify the consequences of individual errors. Finally, the increasing assertion of individual rights in connection with medical care raises the stakes in medical error and reduces social tolerances surrounding medical performance.

Where, then, can we place medical organizations in the spectrum of organizational approaches to error management and reliability? First, we must recognize that in contradiction to the conclusions of the Institute of Medicine and the Quality Interagency Coordination Task Force reports, when it comes to health care, reliability issues are not "much as in any other industry." In fact, only by appreciating the special properties of medical production and medical errors can we hope to arrive at sensible conclusions about promoting medical reliability.

Distinctive Properties of Medical Errors

Medical organizations confront several distinct types of errors. In his study of surgical errors and failures, Charles Bosk (1979) distinguishes between technical, judgmental, normative, and quasi-normative errors. *Technical errors* reflect skill failures. *Judgmental errors* involve the selection of an incorrect strategy of treatment. *Normative errors* occur when the larger social values embedded within medicine as a profession are violated. This error occurs, for example, when a surgeon "has, in the eyes of others, failed to discharge his role obligation conscientiously" (p. 51). *Quasi-normative errors* are failures of subordinates (surgical residents, for instance) to follow the authority of a superior.

Bosk argues that these errors are more socially than objectively defined and determined. He finds that the different kinds of errors are also quite differently treated in surgical organizations. The technical and judgmental errors are frequently subject to fewer preventive efforts or sanctions than the normative ones. Technical and judgmental errors may be taken as inevitable concomitants of learning. As such, they are "forgivable," provided they are not made repetitively by the same person. Normative errors are less forgivable because they reflect a less than reliable commitment on the part of the individual to the norms of the profession. In this sense they threaten the social reputation and, ultimately, acceptance of the profession.

Not only do these distinct kinds of errors occur in surgery but the organizational controls over surgeons are also less powerful than those available in the formal hierarchy that characterizes other organizations. Surgeons, and other doctors, have a significant amount of autonomy in their work. Attending physicians in medical facilities often are not even employees of the facilities in which they operate.

It is now useful to return to the proposition with which this analysis began: successful organizational approaches to reliability are determined both by the properties of the failures an organization seeks to avoid and by the stability of the environmental equilibrium the organization has achieved with respect to those failures. An examination of these two dimensions in relation to medical error can locate medical errors on the organizational reliability continuum laid out earlier.

The failure characteristic, the first dimension, is the boundedness of the failure. Is the failure contained within a narrowly bounded set of variables and people or does it ramify widely outward to threaten elements and people well outside the boundaries of the organization? The second dimension concerns the environmental equilibrium achieved by the organization with respect to its failures. If failures are more or less accepted by the environment, if they do not disturb the fundamental balances in demand or support for organizational activity, then the equilibrium is stable. If failure threatens to change those balances — to undermine social acceptance or prompt the erosion of organizational support or autonomy — then the equilibrium is unstable with respect to failure. Considering these issues together forms the matrix shown in Figure 10.1.

Social Equilibrium with Respect to Failure

Failures	Stable	Unstable
Bounded	Medical treatment organizations	Banks, investment houses, alternative medicine clinics, religious cults
Unbounded	Chemical processing plants, flour mills, oil tankers	Nuclear power plants, air traffic control centers, nuclear weapons agencies

Figure 10.1. Major Reliability Categories for Organizations.

Organizations such as nuclear power plants face the prospect of failures that could well propagate outward to threaten land and people far beyond the reach of the organization. They also stand in precarious relation to environmental support. It's no wonder that the reliability standard imposed on them is that of precluded events.

Chemical processing plants, flour mills, oil tankers, and similar enterprises also face the possibility of failures that could ramify outward from the organization—spreading toxic materials or oil spills into the surrounding environment. But in these cases the environment has accepted the organization and its risks. Chemical plants, refineries, and flour mills do blow up, the effects do literally spill out into their environments, but these organizations generally are allowed to continue their operations. Their managers frequently retain their jobs and continue the trajectory of their careers. The organizations do not suffer dramatically altered public support or a sea change in regulatory requirements. For a variety of reasons, organizations in this category, whatever their history, do not inspire societal dread. Rather, they are steeped in networks of social dependency. This is not to say that the equilibrium they maintain with their environment does not undergo periodic adjustment; they may encounter political, legal, or regulatory pressures for the adoption of new safety technologies, for example. But their trade-offs of reliability for other values, such as market competitiveness, are more or less accepted in society. These organizations are not held to the standard of precluded events. They can build up a cache of acceptance and goodwill based on past performance. The public and organizational managers are satisfied with past records or with gradual reductions in failure rates.

A third category of organizations has core technologies or processes whose failures can threaten the lives or livelihood of organizational members or clients but have little likelihood of propagating beyond that point. Some of these organizations may have unstable and precarious acceptance within their environment, perhaps because a wary public is worried about the harm they may inflict on their own members. A failure, even though it is internal in cause and consequence, may still trigger a public investigation and legal and regulatory incursions and threaten the future of the organization itself. Banks or investment firms, which must manage clients' financial accounts, might fit into this category, also religious cults when their practices result in child abuse, and clinics for alternative medicine. An organizational approach to reliability here may lie in the hiring of external organizations, such as accounting firms, to validate performance or, alternatively, the suppression of information about errors — possibly internally and certainly to the outside world.

Finally, we come to medical organizations. Here again, failures center on the individual patient. Also, the environmental equilibrium that major medical service organizations such as hospitals, clinics, and private physician-run medical corporations establish is resilient to individual treatment errors. As noted, the environment of clients, regulators, and certainly third-party payers allows reliability to be traded off to some measure with cost containment and with speed and efficiency of treatment as well.[4]

Here is one example. A particularly troublesome error among health care workers is a needlestick accident, the penetration of the skin of the worker by a hypodermic needle — generally during or after injecting a patient. Needlesticks expose caregivers to patients' blood, of no small consequence considering that both HIV and hepatitis C viruses can be transmitted in this way. Hospitals, blood banks, and medical testing laboratories have conducted campaigns against needlesticks, ranging from education and training to installing new procedures for disposing of needles. OSHA, the Occupational Health and Safety Administration, has a set of guidelines and recommendations covering needlestick errors.

Yet needlesticks are still a common occurrence in many medical facilities (one hospital averages over one hundred per year). There are now new technologies that can prevent needlesticks—needleless injection systems and self-sheathing needles, although these raise the cost of injections. A HealthCare Worker Needlestick Prevention Act was introduced into the Congress in 1999 mandating the use of these new devices, and four states have passed legislation of their own mandating their use. Yet it is estimated that only 15 percent of hospitals in the United States currently use the new technologies (Bockhold, 2000).

Why do needlestick injuries persist? When the technology is available to prevent these injuries and it is not widely diffused throughout the industry, when it is estimated that 70 percent of needlesticks occur after needle use and that simply following routine disposal procedures could prevent these accidents, and when statistics indicate that experience doesn't reduce the likelihood of needlesticks, it seems reasonable to suspect the existence of values that countervail those of high reliability with respect to this error. What seems likely is that although health care workers and their supervisors are aware of the hazards of a needlestick, they are also aware of the need to get a high volume of patient injections or blood work done within a restricted period of time. Health care managers, institutional boards of directors, and shareholders are interested in keeping medical costs down and speed up. So too are medical insurers, reimbursers, and even patients themselves.

Perhaps the answer to increased reliability with respect to this particular medical error lies less in better training, more careful human factors analysis, new procedures, or closer supervision (some of the "system" factors cited in the IOM report) than it does in a change in the relative distribution of values surrounding the injections and the blood work (safety, efficiency, speed, and convenience), values held not only by those in medical organizations but by the public as well. Changing the relative weights of societal values and demands for reliability is no small task. But these are crucial factors in determining where along the continuum from marginal reliability to precluded events an organization can successfully cast its reliability strategy.

This analysis suggests that an approach to reliability at the level of precluded events is itself precluded for medical organizations. It would take a major shift in public demand or an alteration in the boundedness of medical errors to lay the foundations for such an approach.

In the meantime, the potentially serious, if bounded, nature of medical errors continues to drive reliability strategies in medical organizations. These are currently a mix of formal procedures, relatively uneven managerial supervision (focused primarily on lower-level employees), and extensive trial-and-error training. But another large component in current medical reliability is the professional norms and values of individual medical practitioners. This element keeps medical organizations from lapsing fully into marginal reliability strategies. Indeed one of the major strains in U.S. medicine today is the conflict between the cost-containment values of third-party payers and the reliability norms of individual practitioners. This battle's ultimate result, as a reflection of social tolerances, is more likely than the "systems" design of medical organizations to determine the reliability levels we can attain with respect to medical errors.

Conclusion

What can now be said of the practical implications of this effort to locate medical error within the rubric of reliability theory? What can be done, based on theories of organization, to improve the management of medical error?

First, it is worthwhile to note that just as medical error is overgeneralized when it is seen as similar to error in "any other industry," an error this chapter has tried to undo, we may still be overgeneralizing when we think of medical error generically. There are diverse types of medical error, probably with different properties across medical specialties and medical organizations. Great care must be taken to sort out these types of error and the varying strategies that may be appropriate for each.

This chapter began by noting both the opportunity and the dilemma the IOM report raises with respect to our knowledge about reliability in organized settings. Clearly the report ought to prompt more careful analysis of both the failure properties and environmental tolerances associated with medical reliability. This is not to say that attention to many particular issues in procedures, training, and supervision could not lead to improvements in error statistics throughout medical practice. It is also not to deny the comparatively high levels of reliability already achieved in the medical industry. But simply to import reliability strategies wholesale from other industries is to risk just those systems and design errors the IOM report invoked. Ironically, this approach to medical reliability might turn out to be the greatest medical error of them all.

Notes

1. In addition, one analyst has described *errors of rendition*—actions taken under misperceived or misunderstood definitions of the situation, mental models that guide action that are themselves erroneous (Weick, 1987).

2. For an analysis of this dread, see Wildavsky and Dake (1990), Perrow (1984, chap. 9), and Flynn, J., Slovic, P., & Kunreuther, H. (2001).

3. An insightful analysis of the cognitive requirements for mindfully coping with multiple organizational variables can be found in Weick, Sutcliffe, and Obstfeld (1999).

4. In this respect the role played by malpractice insurance is of interest. It might be viewed as an important component in stabilizing the reliability relationships between medical organizations, their clients, and clients' families.

References

Bockhold, K. (2000). Who's afraid of hepatitis C? *American Journal of Nursing,* 100, 26–31.

Bosk, C. (1979). *Forgive and remember: Managing medical failure.* Chicago: University of Chicago Press.

Flynn, J., Slovic, P., & Kunreuther, H. (Eds.). (2001). *Risk, Media and Stigma.* London: Earthscan Publications.

Kohn, L. T., Corrigan, J. M., & Donaldson, M. S. (Eds.); Committee on Quality of Health Care in America, Institute of Medicine. (2000). *To err is human: Building a safer health system.* Washington, DC: National Academy Press.

LaPorte, T. (1996). High reliability organizations: Unlikely, demanding and at risk. *Journal of Contingencies and Crisis Management, 4,* 60–71.

LaPorte, T., & Consolini, P. (1991). Working in practice but not in theory: Theoretical challenges of high reliability organizations. *Journal of Public Administration Research and Theory, 1,* 19–47.

Perrow, C. (1984). *Normal accidents: Living with high risk technologies.* New York: Basic Books.

Quality Interagency Coordination Task Force. (2000). *Doing what counts for patient safety: Federal actions to reduce medical errors and their impact* (Report of the Quality Interagency Coordination Task Force (QuIC) to the President). Washington, DC: U.S. Government Printing Office.

Roberts, K. (Ed.). (1993). *New challenges to understanding organizations.* New York: Macmillan.

Rochlin, G., & Von Meier, A. (1994). Nuclear power operations: A cross-cultural perspective. *Annual Review of Energy and the Environment, 19,* 153–187.

Sanne, J. (2000). *Creating safety in air traffic control.* Lund, Sweden: Arkiv Forlag.

Schulman, P. (1993a). The analysis of high reliability organizations: A comparative framework. In K. H. Roberts (Ed.), *New challenges to understanding organizations* (pp. 33–53). New York: Macmillan.

Schulman, P. (1993b). The negotiated order of organizational reliability. *Administration and Society, 25,* 353–372.

Schulman, P. (1996). Heroes, organizations and high reliability. *Journal of Contingencies and Crisis Management, 4,* 72–82.

Weick, K. E. (1987). Organizational culture as a source of high reliability. *California Management Review, 29,* 112–127.

Weick, K. E., Sutcliffe, K. M., & Obstfeld, D. (1999). Organizing for high reliability: Processes of collective mindfulness. In B. Staw & R. Sutton (Eds.), *Research in organizational behavior* (Vol. 21, pp. 81–123). Greenwich, CT: JAI.

Wildavsky, A. (1988). *Searching for safety.* New Brunswick, NJ: Transaction.

Wildavsky, A., & Dake, K. (1990). Theories of risk perception: Who fears what and why. *Daedalus, 119*(4), 41–60.

11

Will Airline Safety Models Work in Medicine?

Eric J. Thomas and Robert L. Helmreich

Researchers studying error in medicine (Leape, 1994; Berwick & Leape, 1999) and expert groups (Kohn, Corrigan, & Donaldson, 2000) have suggested that health care providers look to the airline industry as a model for error prevention. However, few published reports critically examine the feasibility of this suggestion. In this chapter, we overview the data sources and training methods used by aviation to monitor and improve safety, discuss their applicability to health care, and report how each has been applied to this domain.

Health care and aviation have important similarities. Pilots and health care providers are highly trained professionals who operate in complex environments where teams interact with technology. In both domains, risk varies from low to high, with threats coming from a variety of sources in the environment. Safety is a superordinate goal for both professions, but cost issues influence the commitment of resources for safety efforts. When error is suspected, litigation and increased regulatory oversight are threats in both professions.

The medical venues where parallels with aviation have been explored most fully are the operating room and the emergency room. In both, team coordination and interaction are required to accomplish multiple tasks. Helmreich and Merritt (1998) have examined aspects of the professional cultures of pilots and of doctors working in the operating room (anesthesiologists and surgeons). Using questionnaires with comparable content, they found similarities between the cultures in both positive and negative values. Positively, both groups are proud of being members of an elite professional group that requires extensive training and selective qualification. Negatively, both pilots and doctors tend to deny personal vulnerability, endorsing items indicating that their decision making is as good in emergencies as under normal conditions, that they can leave behind personal problems when working, and that their performance is not degraded by working with inexperienced personnel. (A significant percentage of doctors also deny the deleterious effects of fatigue on performance.) These aspects of professional culture have implications for patient and aircraft safety. Professional pride motivates individuals to do their best, but the perception of invulnerability may reduce perceptions of the need for teamwork and for the practice of countermeasures against error.

However, there are also major differences between health care and aviation. Aircraft accidents are infrequent, highly visible, and often involve massive loss of life. And in stark contrast to health care, this loss of life may include the lives of the aviation professionals themselves. Aircraft accidents result in exhaustive investigation into causal factors, public reports, and remedial action. Medical errors and the subsequent adverse events happen to individual patients and seldom receive national publicity. More important, there is no standardized method of investigation, documentation, and dissemination of findings—despite the recent report by the Institute of Medicine that estimated between 44,000 (Thomas et al., 1999) and 98,000 (Leape, Lawthers, Brennan, & Johnson, 1993) annual deaths from medical error.

Normal operations in each profession are also quite different. Training in medicine is longer than in aviation and involves significant amounts of hands-on learning, whereas aviation relies on simulation to train pilots and maintain their skills. Pilots' professional skills (now including teamwork as well as technical abilities) are formally evaluated on a regular basis (at a minimum, annually), and failure to pass can lead to loss of licensure. Medicine's means of ensuring competence are less stringent and less explicit, and medicine seems more tolerant of such behavior (Stewart, 1999). Sociologists have identified several methods used by the medical profession to deal with incompetence. They include quiet chats in the hallway, protective support, diversion of patients (Rosenthal, 1995), withdrawing favors, talking in an educational manner, confrontation by committee, and referring difficult cases to administrators (Freidson, 1970). Although incompetence and negligence contribute to a minority of the errors and adverse events in medicine, they should be addressed more explicitly, perhaps in ways modeled in part on the aviation model.

Another difference between the professions is that patients are more complex than airplanes, and their health is influenced by numerous factors, such as socioeconomic status, access to health care, and genetic determinants. The information needed to care for patients is also more complex because it changes so fast. New technologies appear and are implemented more rapidly in medicine than in aviation.

Furthermore, a cockpit crew is an easily defined team with a formal hierarchy of authority that makes decisions during a flight that has a clear beginning and end. One of us (Robert Helmreich) sparked an acrimonious debate when speaking to an audience of anesthesiologists and surgeons by asking, "Who is in charge in the operating room?" Each group argued passionately for its authority. A health care team may include social workers, lab technicians, nurses, students, doctors, and others who are working from disparate locations to care for a patient over days, months, or even years.

However, the complexity of the medical environment does not by itself prevent the applicability of aviation safety methods to health care. It does mean that adaptation of aviation safety methods should be done with care, and as discussed in the remainder of this chapter, a great deal of progress in this area has already been made.

The Aviation Approach to Safety

The aviation industry and regulators have found a number of ways to collect pertinent error data, with a view to managing error.

Sources of Error Data in Aviation

As mentioned earlier, one primary source of information in aviation is the in-depth investigation of accidents and incidents. However, the most valuable source of safety information is the assessment of normal operations, a data source vastly underused in health care. The airline industry uses multiple sources of data for normal process monitoring. Quick access data recorders provide analysts with the same categories of information available to accident investigators, in a program known as Flight Operations Quality Assurance (FOQA). Data from every flight of aircraft equipped with the recorders are analyzed for events that exceed predefined flight parameters (for example, unstable approaches).

FOQA data provide highly accurate information about *what* occurs during a flight, but they do not indicate *why* these things happen. So confidential surveys of pilots and other crew members are used to learn about perceptions of organizational commitment to safety and attitudes about teamwork, leadership, and error. This focus on crew survey data stems from a National Aeronautics and Space Administration (NASA) study in the late 1970s that found that more than 70 percent of airline accidents were the result not of mechanical failure or weather but of such interpersonal aspects of flying an aircraft as leadership, communication, decision making, and shared awareness of the situation (Helmreich & Foushee, 1993).

In response to the NASA study, Helmreich and colleagues developed the Cockpit Management Attitudes Questionnaire (CMAQ) (Helmreich, 1984) to measure crew attitudes about communication, teamwork, and leadership. Subsequently, a revised instrument, the Flight Management Attitudes Questionnaire (FMAQ), incorporated the CMAQ and extended its coverage to address organizational issues and dimensions of national culture that contribute to error (Helmreich & Merritt, 1998). Helmreich and colleagues have administered the CMAQ or FMAQ to 40,000 pilots from over forty airlines and twenty-five countries. The questionnaire is reliable, responsive to changes in attitudes that occur after training (Gregorich, Helmreich, & Wilhelm, 1990), and predicts the quality of crew teamwork (Foushee, 1984; Helmreich, Foushee, Benson, & Russini, 1986; Helmreich, Wilhelm, Gregorich, & Chidester, 1990). Training designed to instill or enhance attitudes associated with error reduction in flight crew members (discussed in more detail later) has improved safety-related attitudes and behavior (Helmreich & Wilhelm, 1991) and is now mandated by the International Civil Aviation Organization (ICAO), the United Nations organization that regulates international airline traffic.

Nonpunitive, incident reporting systems are a third data source used by aviation (Wiener & Nagel, 1989). Several countries have national aviation incident reporting systems in which organizations and individuals can report an adverse event without having their identity connected to it. In the United States the new Aviation Safety Action Partnership (ASAP) (Federal Aviation Administration, 2000) permits pilots to report incidents to their own companies with the same limited immunity provided by the national Aviation Safety Reporting System (ASRS) (Reynard, 1986), thus allowing companies to take immediate corrective action. Funded by the Federal Aviation Administration (FAA) and administered independently by NASA, ASRS receives over 30,000 reports per year and issues alerts to the FAA and airlines. ASRS does not recommend corrective actions, and both individual reporters and the associated airline are kept anonymous. In contrast, because ASAP reports are made to the respondent's own company and because the data are airline specific, it is easier for an airline to use these data to identify problems and take corrective actions.

Because incident reports are voluntary, they cannot provide baseline rates of risk and error. This creates particular difficulties for

Table 11.1. Categories of Error During Normal Flight.

1. Violation	Conscious failure to adhere to procedures or regulations *Example: Performing a checklist from memory*
2. Procedural	Followed procedures with wrong execution *Example: Wrong altitude setting dialed into the MCP*
3. Communication	Missing or incorrect information exchange or mis-interpretation of communication *Example: Misunderstood altitude clearance*
4. Proficiency	Error due to a lack of knowledge or skill *Example: Inability to program automation*
5. Decision	Discretionary crew decision that unnecessarily increases risk *Example: Unnecessary navigation through adverse weather*

decision makers when allocating resources, because they do not know whether an incident report represents a common problem or a once-in-a-lifetime event (March, Sproull, & Tamuz, 1991). In addition, incident-reporting systems cannot be used to determine whether certain events are increasing or decreasing in frequency after an intervention.

A fourth source of data about error in aviation is an observational methodology that has been under development for over fifteen years by the University of Texas Human Factors Research Project. The Line Operations Safety Audit (LOSA) places expert observers in the cockpit during normal flights to record threats to safety, errors and their management, and behaviors identified as critical in preventing accidents. This approach is supported by the FAA and the ICAO (Helmreich, Wilhelm, Klinect, & Merritt, in press), and confidential data have been collected on more than 3,800 domestic and international airline flights. LOSA results verify the ubiquity of threat and error in the aviation environment, with an average of two threats and two errors observed per flight (Klinect, Wilhelm, & Helmreich, 1999). Table 11.1 lists and defines the five basic error types empirically observed, and Figure 11.1 illustrates the relative frequency of each type of error.

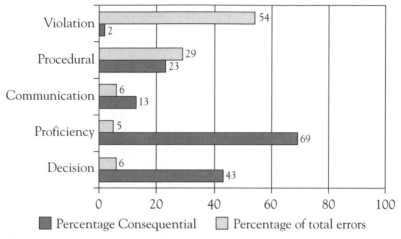

Figure 11.1. Percentages of Each Type of Error and Consequential Errors.

This error classification is useful because different interventions are required to prevent and mitigate different types of error. Proficiency errors suggest technical training is needed, whereas communication and decision errors call for team training. Procedural errors may result from human limitations or from procedures that are inadequate and need change. Violations may stem from a culture of noncompliance, perceptions of invulnerability, or poor procedures. That more than half of observed errors were violations was unexpected. This lack of compliance found by LOSA is a source of concern that has triggered internal reviews of procedures and organizational cultures. Figure 11.1 also shows what percentage of each kind of error was classified as consequential, that is, resulting in such undesired events as near misses, navigational deviation, or additional error. Although the overall percentages of proficiency and decision errors are low, these errors have the highest probability of being consequential (Klinect, 1999). Even nonconsequential errors increase risk: teams that violate procedures are 1.6 times more likely than other teams to commit other types of errors (Helmreich, 1999). In sum, direct observation methods such as LOSA provide crucial information about error that would be otherwise unavailable, and that leads to specific interventions appropriate to the type of errors identified.

Managing Error in Aviation

Given that these data sources reveal the ubiquity of threat and error, one key to safety is the effective management of these ubiquitous events. *Simulation* training and *crew resource management* (CRM) training (Helmreich, 1999) are two methods used in aviation to manage error. CRM has been a major change in training that had previously addressed only technical aspects of flying. It addresses human performance limiters such as fatigue and stress, examines the nature of human error, and defines behaviors that are error countermeasures, such as leadership, briefings, monitoring and cross-checking, decision making, and review and modification of plans. CRM is now required for flight crews worldwide, and data support its effectiveness in changing attitudes and behavior and in enhancing safety (Helmreich & Wilhelm, 1991). Two important conclusions emerge from evaluations of CRM training: first, it needs to be ongoing, because attitudes and practices decay in the absence of recurrent training and reinforcement, and second, it needs to be tailored to conditions and experience within individual organizations (Klinect et al., 1999).

Simulation also plays an important role in training cockpit crew members. Sophisticated simulators allow full crews to practice dealing with error-inducing situations under nonjeopardous conditions and to receive feedback on both their individual and team performance. Line Oriented Flight Training (LOFT), developed in conjunction with CRM, provides challenging scenarios in which full crews can practice the behaviors taught in CRM. The integration of simulation and CRM has been a critical element in dealing with the interpersonal aspects of flight management.

Applications to Medical Error

Three key aviation data sources (surveys, incident reports, and direct observation) have been used in health care, as have simulation and CRM. In this section, we offer examples of their use and discuss their strengths and limitations when applied to health care.

Surveys

We have adapted the FMAQ survey used in aviation and administered it to 1,033 medical personnel working in teaching and nonteaching hospitals in the United States, Israel, Germany, Switzerland, and Italy to measure their attitudes about stress, teamwork, and error. The results are enlightening, especially when compared to survey data from over 30,000 cockpit crew members. Pilots were least likely to deny the effects of fatigue on performance (26 percent) when compared with surgical attendings (70 percent) and anesthesia attendings (47 percent). The denial of fatigue and its effects on performance may help individuals adapt to the rigors of medical training, but a healthy recognition of how fatigue affects performance reduces the likelihood of error and increases the use of threat and error management strategies (Helmreich & Merritt, 1998).

More pilots (97 percent) and ICU personnel (94 percent) reject steep authority hierarchies (those in which senior team members are not open to input from junior team members) when compared with anesthesia attendings (85 percent) and surgical attendings (55 percent). A relatively large number of surgical attendings and residents gave high ratings to the teamwork they experienced with other surgical attendings (64 to 73 percent reported high levels of teamwork, and 7 to 9 percent reported low levels) compared with anesthesia residents, anesthesia nurses, and surgical nurses (10 to 28 percent reported high levels of teamwork, and 39 to 47 percent reported low levels). Acceptance of steep authority hierarchies within teams and differing perceptions of the level of teamwork among team members are attitudes that may predispose a team to commit errors and decrease the team's ability to trap and mitigate error.

Responding to questions about medical error, only one out of three medical personnel reported that errors are handled appropriately at his or her hospital. A third of ICU respondents did not acknowledge that they make errors. More than half of the ICU respondents reported that they find it difficult to discuss mistakes and said that barriers to discussing error included personal reputation, job security, the high expectations of society, sanctions from licensing boards, and the threat of malpractice suits.

Health care organizations can use a survey like this as one component of a safety program because it mines data from the "front lines" that may be otherwise unavailable. Further, surveys are relatively inexpensive to administer. Among their limitations, however, are the difficulty of getting high response rates from health care providers and the absence of research demonstrating a link between attitudes and behavior.

Incident Reporting

Numerous incident reporting systems exist in health care. But compared to systems of the airline industry, these systems are relatively immature and their effects not well evaluated. Barach and Small (2000) note that incident reporting systems exist in anesthesia, emergency medicine, intensive care, transfusion medicine, cytology, occupational and industrial medicine, cardiac surgery, pharmacy, and nursing. The Veterans Administration just announced a national near-miss reporting system, to be operated in conjunction with the National Aeronautics and Space Administration ("VA Plans No-Penalty Medical Error Reporting," 2000), and the Joint Commission on Accreditation of Healthcare Organizations (1998) requires hospitals to have reporting systems and to conduct root cause analyses of certain events. In addition, several states have medical adverse incident reporting systems (Kohn et al., 2000).

Although the Institute of Medicine report on medical error strongly recommended both mandatory and voluntary reporting systems, there is little evidence of these systems' effectiveness and much concern that the reports might lead to medical malpractice lawsuits (Brennan, 2000). As in aviation, incident data provided through self-reports are limited because they cannot be used to establish an accurate estimate of the baseline incidence of events — information that is crucial in health care when making decisions to allocate scarce resources and when evaluating the effects of interventions. Nevertheless, the aviation industry overcame similar fears of litigation, and reporting systems are currently believed to be one of that industry's most important sources of data for preventing error.

Direct Observation

The operating room has been the primary site where health care organizations have applied safety methods from aviation. This milieu is more complex than the cockpit, with differing specialties interacting to treat a patient whose condition and response may have unknown characteristics (Helmreich & Schaefer, 1994). In contrast, aircraft tend to be more predictable than patients. Despite these differences and legal and cultural barriers to the disclosure of error, we have observed operations and noted instances of suboptimal teamwork and communication paralleling those found in the cockpit (Helmreich & Schaefer, 1994). These are behaviors addressed in CRM training.

Andrews et al. (1997) observed surgical teams during rounds and other routine activities and found that 17.7 percent of patients admitted to a surgical service in a Chicago teaching hospital suffered at least one *serious* adverse event, meaning that the patient suffered at least temporary physical disability. Several other investigators have videotaped trauma resuscitations as a method of measuring errors and quality of care. According to analysis of such videotapes, errors during trauma resuscitation are common, due to high-level task complexity (Xiao et al., 1996). Trauma resuscitation involves multiple and concurrent tasks, uncertainty, changing plans, compressed work procedures, and high workloads. Many of the errors observed were due to poor teamwork. Analysis of videotapes of intubations during trauma resuscitation attributed eight of twenty-eight errors to poor teamwork (MacKenzie et al., 1996). Other reviews of such tapes identified interpersonal problems among team members (Townsend, Clark, Ramenofsky, & Diamond, 1993); deficiencies in leadership (Santora, Trooskin, Blank, Clarke, & Schinco, 1996), including poor communication with team members (Sugrue, Seger, Kerridge, Sloane, & Deane, 1995); and lack of team member adherence to assigned responsibilities (Hoyt et al., 1988; Michaelson & Levi, 1997).

Limitations to direct observation in health care include the resources and personnel time it requires and concerns that plaintiffs' attorneys could be given legal access to the data and that organizations might use the data in compiling job performance ratings. However, with well-trained observers looking for explicit, measurable events and with appropriate attention paid to hindsight bias (Fischoff, 1975) and other subtleties of measuring human performance (Cook & Woods, 1994), direct observation of care can discover invaluable opportunities for improvement.

Simulation

Lifelike patient simulators have been developed, with general anesthesia simulators leading the way (Gaba & DeAnda, 1988; Kapur & Steadmen, 1998). The complexity of simulating the entire operating room environment is a challenge, but one that will likely be overcome with improved technology and investment. Trauma simulators are also being developed (Small et al., 1999), as are simulators for simpler procedures such as flexible sigmoidoscopy (Tuggy, 1998). Although incorporating simulation into medical training and continuing education certainly makes sense, its impact upon the practice of medicine has yet to be demonstrated.

Crew Resource Management in Health Care

The general idea of applying CRM to medicine certainly has face validity, and health care organizations should pursue further research in the area. As we described earlier, CRM addresses human performance limiters such as fatigue and stress, examines the nature of human error, and teaches behaviors that are error countermeasures, such as leadership, briefings, monitoring and cross-checking, decision making, and review and modification of plans.

Although it is not known exactly which CRM behaviors are correlated with error in medicine, researchers have directed significant effort to interventions with CRM-type team training programs, primarily in the emergency room setting. This effort is led by scientists from Dynamics Research Corporation (DRC). DRC has developed a training program for emergency department teams and is testing its effectiveness in a group of eleven military and civilian hospitals ("Bringing Cutting-Edge 'MedTeams' Concepts to Your ED," 1999; National Health Policy Forum, 1999). CRM concepts have also been incorporated into anesthesia simulation (Weinger et al., 1994) and trauma simulation (Small et al., 1999).

The application of CRM to health care does seem to make sense, but we advise a cautious approach, beginning with using focus groups and survey data to understand what CRM attitudes and behaviors appear to be important in health care, then using observational data to identify the most important CRM-related behaviors, and finally, developing a CRM training program and evaluating it in a well-designed clinical trial.

Conclusion

There are differences between health care and aviation, but similarities also abound, and there is a great opportunity for all of us in health care to learn from aviation. The medical field is adopting the aviation industry's approach to monitoring error by using incident reports, survey data, and direct observation. Medicine is just now learning how to implement these methods for monitoring error in patient care. Their usefulness in actually reducing error and improving patient safety is promising but far from proven. For example, there is no research available even to inform the basic design of incident reporting systems. We need to study how events are defined, how the data are gathered and analyzed, and how they are used to make decisions. Consider, for example, that those implementing incident reporting systems should know that the way people define events reflects their understanding of those events and shapes how organizations respond to them. Tamuz (2000) studied seven safety information systems and found that these systems classified potential dangers either as threats to rule enforcement or as opportunities for learning. Each of these differing categorizations subsequently influenced the construction of an information gathering system and what that system was designed to collect. Other trade-offs exist in the ways we choose to collect and analyze data, and these should be explored as more incident reporting systems are implemented.

Simulation and crew resource management, aviation's methods of preventing and managing error, are being studied in detail in anesthesia and emergency medicine, and research may soon demonstrate the decreases in error we all hope for. Certainly, medical personnel would benefit from feedback on their performance, including interpersonal skills.

As the aviation safety methods garner more attention in medicine, it is to be hoped they will be applied in a thoughtful manner. Given the pressure to improve patient safety, health care organizations may begin to adopt the aviation approach blindly, without the necessary research. Ideally, well-designed, multidisciplinary research published in peer-reviewed journals will inform our application of these methods to health care.

References

Andrews, L. B., Stocking, C., Krizek, T., Gottlieb, L., Krizek, C., Vargish, T., & Siegler, M. (1997, February 1). An alternative strategy for studying adverse events in medical care. *Lancet, 349,* 309–313.

Barach, P., & Small, S. D. (2000). Reporting and preventing medical mishaps: Lessons from non-medical near miss reporting systems. *British Medical Journal, 320,* 759–763.

Berwick, D. M., & Leape, L. L. (1999). Reducing errors in medicine. *British Medical Journal, 319,* 136–137.

Brennan, T. A. (2000). The Institute of Medicine report on medical errors: Could it do harm? *New England Journal of Medicine, 342,* 1123–1125.

Bringing cutting-edge "MedTeams" concepts to your ED: Novel program eliminates errors, cuts liability risks. (1999, March). *ED Management, 11,* 25–29.

Cook, R. I., & Woods, D. D. (1994). Operating at the sharp end: The complexity of human error. In M. S. Bogner (Ed.), *Human error in medicine* (pp. 255–310). Mahway, NJ: Erlbaum.

Federal Aviation Administration. (2001). *Aviation safety action programs* (Advisory Circular 120–66A). Washington, DC: Author.

Fischoff, B. (1975). Hindsight does not equal foresight: The effect of outcome knowledge on judgment under uncertainty. *Journal of Experimental Psychology, 1,* 288–299.

Foushee, H. C. (1984). Dyads and triads at 25,000 feet: Factors affecting group process and aircrew performance. *American Psychologist, 39,* 885–993.

Freidson, E. (1970). *The profession of medicine: A study of the sociology of applied knowledge.* New York: HarperCollins.

Gaba, D. M., & DeAnda, A. A. (1988). A comprehensive anesthesia simulation environment: Recreating the operating room for research and training. *Anesthesiology, 69,* 387–396.

Gregorich, S. E., Helmreich, R. L., & Wilhelm, J. A. (1990). The structure of cockpit management attitudes. *Journal of Applied Psychology, 75,* 682–690.

Helmreich, R. L. (1984). Cockpit management attitudes. *Human Factors, 26,* 583–589.

Helmreich, R. L. (1999). *Culture and error in safety in aviation: The management commitment.* London: Royal Aeronautical Society.

Helmreich, R. L., & Foushee, H. C. (1993). Why crew resource management: Empirical and theoretical bases of human factors training in aviation.

In E. L. Wiener, B. G. Kanki, & R. L. Helmreich (Eds.), *Cockpit resource management* (pp. 3–45). New York: Academic Press.

Helmreich, R. L., Foushee, H. C., Benson, R., & Russini, W. (1986). Cockpit management attitudes: Exploring the attitude-behavior linkage. *Aviation, Space, and Environmental Medicine, 57,* 1198–1200.

Helmreich, R. L., & Merritt, A. C. (1998). *Culture at work: National, organizational and professional influences.* Aldershot, UK: Ashgate.

Helmreich, R. L., & Schaefer, H. G. (1994). Team performance in the operating room. In M. S. Bogner (Ed.), *Human error in medicine* (pp. 225–253). Mahway, NJ: Erlbaum.

Helmreich, R. L., & Wilhelm, J. A. (1991). Outcomes of crew resource management training. *International Journal of Aviation Psychology, 1,* 287–300.

Helmreich, R. L., Wilhelm, J. A., Gregorich, S. E., & Chidester, T. R. (1990). Preliminary results from the evaluation of cockpit resource management training: Performance ratings of flight crews. *Aviation, Space, and Environmental Medicine, 61,* 576–579.

Helmreich, R. L., Wilhelm, J. A., Klinect, J. R., & Merritt, A. C. (in press). Culture, error and crew resource management. In E. Salas, C. A. Bowers, & E. Edens (Eds.), *Improving teamwork in organizations: Applications of resource management* (pp. 305–331). Mahway, NJ: Erlbaum.

Hoyt, D. B., Shackford, S. R., Freidland, P. H., Mackersie, R. C., Hansbrough, J. F., Wachtel, T. L., & Fortune, J. B. (1988). Video recording trauma resuscitations: An effective teaching technique. *Journal of Trauma, 28,* 435–440.

Joint Commission on Accreditation of Healthcare Organizations. (1998, May 1). *Sentinel Event Alert,* No. 3.

Kapur, P. A., & Steadmen, R. H. (1998). Patient simulator competency testing: Ready for takeoff. *Anesthesia and Analgesia, 86,* 1157–1159.

Klinect, J. R., Wilhelm, J. A., & Helmreich, R. L. (1999). Threat and error management: Data from line operations safety audits. In R. S. Jensen (Ed.), *Proceedings of the Tenth International Symposium on Aviation Psychology* (pp. 683–688). Columbus: Ohio State University.

Kohn, L. T., Corrigan, J. M., & Donaldson, M. S. (Eds.); Committee on Quality of Health Care in America, Institute of Medicine. (2000). *To err is human: Building a safer health system.* Washington, DC: National Academy Press.

Leape, L. L. (1994). Error in medicine. *Journal of the American Medical Association, 272,* 1851–1857.

Leape, L. L., Lawthers, A. G., Brennan, T. A., & Johnson, W. G. (1993, May). The preventability of medical injury. *Quality Review Bulletin,* 144–149.

MacKenzie, C. F., Jeffries, N. J., Hunter, W. A., Bernhard, W. N., Xiao, Y., & the

LOTAS Group. (1996). Comparison of self-reporting of deficiencies in airway management with video analysis of actual performance. *Human Factors, 38,* 623–635.

March, J. G., Sproull, L. S., & Tamuz, M. (1991). Learning from samples of one or fewer. *Organizational Science, 2,* 1–3.

Michaelson, M., & Levi, L. (1997). Videotaping in the admitting area: A most useful tool for quality improvement of the trauma care. *European Journal of Emergency Medicine, 4,* 94–96.

National Health Policy Forum. (1999, May 14). *Reducing medical error: Can you be as safe in a hospital as you are in a jet?* (Issue Brief). Washington, DC: Georgetown University.

Reynard, W. D., Billings, C. E., Cheaney, E. S., & Hardy, R. (1986). *The development of the NASA Aviation Safety Reporting System* (NASA Reference Publication 1114). Springfield, VA: National Aeronautics and Space Administration, Scientific and Technical Information Branch.

Rosenthal, M. M. (1995). *The incompetent doctor: Behind closed doors.* Bristol, PA: Open University Press.

Santora, T. A., Trooskin, S. Z., Blank, C. A., Clarke, J. R., & Schinco, M. A. (1996). Video assessment of trauma response: Adherence to ATLS protocols. *American Journal of Emergency Medicine, 14,* 564–569.

Small, S. D., Wuerz, R. C., Simon, R., Shapiro, N., Conn, A., & Setnik, G. (1999). Demonstration of high-fidelity simulation team training for emergency medicine. *Academic Emergency Medicine, 6,* 312–323.

Stewart, J. B. (1999). *Blind eye: How the medical establishment let a doctor get away with murder.* New York: Simon & Schuster.

Sugrue, M., Seger, M., Kerridge, R., Sloane, D., & Deane, S. (1995). A prospective study of the performance of the trauma team leader. *Journal of Trauma, 38,* 79–82.

Tamuz, M. (2000). Defining away dangers: A study in the influence of managerial cognition on information systems. In T. Lant & Z. Shapira (Eds.), *Managerial and organizational cognition.* Mahway, NJ: Erlbaum.

Thomas, E. J., Studdert, D. M., Newhouse, J. P., Zbar, B.I.W., Howard, K. M., Williams, E. J., & Brennan, T. A. (1999). Costs of medical injuries in Colorado and Utah in 1992. *Inquiry, 36,* 255–264.

Townsend, R. N., Clark, R., Ramenofsky, M. L., & Diamond, D. L. (1993). ATLS-based videotape trauma resuscitation review: Education and outcome. *Journal of Trauma, 34,* 133–138.

Tuggy, M. L. (1998). Virtual reality flexible sigmoidoscopy simulator training: Impact on resident performance. *Journal of the American Board of Family Practice, 11,* 426–433.

VA plans no-penalty medical error reporting. (2000, May 31). *New York Times*,
    p. A21.
Weinger, M. B., Herndon, O. W., Zornow, M. H., Paulus, M. P., Gaba, D. M.,
    and Dallen, L. T. (1994). An objective methodology for task analysis and
    workload assessment in anesthesia providers. *Anesthesiology, 80*(1), 77–92.
Wiener, E., & Nagel, D. (1989). *Human factors in aviation.* New York: Academic
    Press.
Xiao, Y., Hunter, W. A., Mackenzie, C. F., Jeffries, N. J., Horst, R. L., & the
    LOTAS Group. (1996). Task complexity in emergency medical care and
    its implications for team coordination. *Human Factors, 38,* 636–645.

Part Five

Where Do We Go from Here?

The chapters in Part Four were authored by organization theo-
rists. Organization scholars are relatively new to the study of
medical error. Of course research on medical error has a long history in professional medicine, sociology, and human factors engineering. Still, few efforts have been made to integrate insights from
these separate domains into a conceptual whole. We envisaged that
this book would provide a small step in this direction, and we take
that step in Part Five, which comprises Chapter Twelve.

The chapter begins by summarizing the insights and implications generated by the authors of the chapters presented in Parts
One through Four. It then draws out a number of themes that are
critical both for understanding what we in health care know about
medical errors and for understanding what we do now. The chapter highlights the need to understand the culture of medicine—how
doctors are socialized into the profession and how they think about
their work—and the necessity of including doctors as key stakeholders in any process of deriving organizational and systemic solutions to this important problem. It draws attention to impediments
to defining errors and shows how our understanding of medical errors is shaped by the context in which we find ourselves. It illustrates the central role of medical uncertainty and how uncertainty

is, perversely, the one certainty in the practice of medicine. Then, taking all these things into account, this concluding chapter suggests an agenda for future action, research, and education.

12

Struggling to Understand, Struggling to Act

Marilynn M. Rosenthal and Kathleen M. Sutcliffe

What is remarkable about the Institute of Medicine (IOM) report *To Err Is Human* is that such a flawed document could become such a powerful force for action.

Perhaps this was the major intention of the IOM Committee on Quality of Health Care in America. The report itself merits scrutiny, particularly of the data on which it is based. It is essential now to move beyond this report's limited scope and to understand medical mistakes from a variety of perspectives, many of which are presented in this book and summed up in this chapter. Contrary to the report's tacit allegation, myriad efforts to address medical mistakes have been in place for some time. We need to think more about them. In addition to closer scrutiny of the industry approaches to error reduction touted in the report, it is essential for us to arrive at a deeper understanding of the medical profession's culture of work and how that culture of uncertainty influences what doctors classify as mistakes. Finally, this concluding chapter addresses prospects for new research and action agendas.

The Institute of Medicine Report

To Err Is Human (Kohn, Corrigan, & Donaldson, 2000) unleashed a dramatic reaction in the media, in the government, and in the health care professions on its release in December 1999. It made headlines in newspapers, TV and radio newscasts, and professional newsletters across the country. Comparing the number of deaths occurring in U.S. hospitals because of medical mistakes to the number of deaths that would result from two jumbo jets crashing each day made a graphic impression on the general public. It shone a public spotlight on problems the medical profession has been struggling with for decades.

The report has produced profound external pressure on the profession of medicine, health care organizations, and the health care system. Mass media, the White House, Congress, governmental agencies, those who pay the medical care bills, and consumers were and are aroused. In this, the IOM report has been a success. As a thoughtful, consistently reliable and accurate analysis, it leaves a lot to be desired. And as Paul Schulman suggests (in Chapter Ten), it may itself constitute a *medical error*.

The IOM report demands action without considering realities; it uses data without careful analysis; it promotes models without evidence; it sets unrealistic deadlines; it fails to mention the resources needed to mount action; it suggests use of technology whose reliability is untested. Most worrisome, it minimizes the organizational and cultural barriers to change in the medical profession and in the health care institutions where patient care is delivered. The report acknowledges that a comprehensive approach to patient safety is needed (Kohn et al., 2000, p. 3). It also notes and then brushes aside the formidable outside barriers of cost pressures, liability restraints, and resistance to change and pays insufficient attention to other seemingly insurmountable barriers, such as highly fragmented delivery systems.

It urges the corporations who are the biggest payers of health care benefits to contract only with providers who will meet requirements for particular activities: mandatory error reporting systems, computerized physician order-entry systems (PCOES), and a 50 percent error reduction in five years. Each of these items, along with other recommended activities, although clearly important, has serious problems. It is impossible to implement a mandatory reporting system. PCOES are not only expensive but also rife with technological and human problems. It is difficult to establish a deadline for error reduction when few reliable baseline data on error incidence are available.

The IOM report as a political document has been a huge success. It generated a flurry of reaction from the White House as the president called for a national mandatory reporting system, ordered the Health Care Financing Administration (HCFA) (now the Centers for Medicare and Medicaid Services [CMS]) to set new error reduction standards for Medicare payments, and demanded that the three hundred provider groups competing for the Federal Employees Health Benefits program meet such standards. Congressional committees called hearings in preparation for legislative action. Big corporate payers of health benefits formed the Leapfrog Group, which has made its own demands for error reduction. The message to the public has been one of concern and concerted action. Then reality set in. It is that reality this book addresses.

The president backed off his demand for a national mandatory reporting system, Congressional hearings have been put on hold, and the Leapfrog Group is now gathering better information before it formalizes its demands.

Despite all the criticisms leveled in the previous paragraphs, a debt is owed to the IOM committee. *To Err is Human*—along with the more recently released *Crossing the Quality Chasm* (Committee on Quality of Health Care in America, 2001)—is the latest and most powerful pressure from the outside continually needed to prod the profession of medicine into renewed action. Doctors, nurses, and hospitals have always been concerned about patient safety, about medical mistakes and adverse events. Nevertheless, they, like all professions and organizations, get stuck in old ways of looking at their work. Jolts, jabs, and judgments from the outside are regularly needed to bring renewed energy and new determination. The IOM report certainly brings that.

What is needed now is to proceed forward to thoughtful, objective, and sustained analysis and understanding of facts, data, and their limitations. Furthermore, we must seek understanding of the multiple perspectives and current efforts in place, of the realistic applicability of new error reduction concepts from other industries, and of the challenging barriers to cultural and organizational change that lie ahead.

So, what do we think we know? What do we think we do? What can we do better?

What Do We Know? How Reliable Are the Data?

David Studdert, Troyen Brennan, and Eric Thomas, in the lead chapter in this book, provide one of the most thoughtful and thorough critiques available of two major sources of data on medical mistakes: the Harvard Medical Practice Study (HMPS) (Brennan et al., 1991) and the replication of the Harvard study in Utah and Colorado (UCMPS) (Thomas et al., 2000), for both of which they were among the principal investigators. These two seminal U.S. studies looked at all *adverse events* in a sample of hospital admissions in each of three states for a single year and determined which were negligent. The New York study built on the Medical Insurance Feasibility Study (MIFS) led by Don Harper Mills (1978) to measure rates of injury in hospitalized patients in California. The MIFS found a 4.6 percent adverse event (AE) rate; the 1990 HMPS a 3.7 percent AE rate, and the 1992 UCMPS a 2.9 percent AE rate.

Studdert, Brennan, and Thomas point out that certain findings are similar across all the studies they discuss. Operating room events are a major cause of AEs; one-half of AEs take place in the emergency room (ER), and a high percentage of the ER adverse events are negligent. These authors also point to the major problems found in prescribing, filling, and administering medications. These findings explain some of the recommendation for action of the IOM report.

Studdert and his colleagues also point to Ross Wilson's Quality in Australian Health Care Study (Wilson et al., 1995), which used the Harvard methodology and found a 16.6 percent AE rate overall. And they also mention the Andrews et al. (1997) study from the University of Chicago, which found a 17.7 percent AE rate in one university teaching hospital. (But as Studdert, Brennan, and Thomas note, the Andrews study and UCMPS differed dramatically in sampling and other aspects of methodology, which may limit their comparability.)

Studdert, Brennan, and Thomas wisely point out the enormous methodological problems in all these studies. The U.S. and Australian studies depend on record review, despite the fact that medical records are notoriously incomplete and therefore unreliable. They also point out that teams of reviewers often disagreed on the definition of an adverse event. This is an important observation that will be addressed further along in this chapter. In addition these authors note that the conditions of health care delivery changed over the three decades during which data were gathered for the three medical practice studies looked at in detail (data were gathered in the 1970s for the MIFS, the HMPS looked at records from 1984, and the UCMPS examined records from 1992). Managed care and other market and regulatory dynamics intervened during this period, limiting comparability among the three.

The key insights to be gained here are that medical error data collection is done in a dynamic and changing field; that there is no uniform definition of an adverse event, error, or mistake, negligent or not, preventable or not; and that state-of-the-art studies are finding different results. And that state-of-the-art is really a Model T Ford, to use a Michigan metaphor. The implication is that researchers and policymakers should be judicious in using the data and in drawing conclusions. There is a great deal more work to do.

In this health care era dominated by cost containment, Studdert and his colleagues offer an economic analysis of the cost of AEs. According to their calculations, the costs are staggering. In New

York, $2.8 billion was spent on treatment necessitated by AEs in the hospitals; in Utah and Colorado, $661.9 million. These calculations do not include various costs to patients and their families.

Further, these authors go on to link their findings with the exigencies of the tort system. They discover that the overwhelming majority of patients suffering an AE deemed negligent by these studies do not sue. This is an important condemnation of the effectiveness of the tort system, which neither deters nor compensates equitably. The tort system is a social mechanism that suggests justice and recompense. It does not, in general, deliver on that suggestion (Rosenthal, 1987) and may complicate efforts to establish effective error reporting systems.

The implication of these findings is important to the major thrust of this book. As Studdert, Brennan, and Thomas point out, error prevention strategies such as error reporting systems hinge on the free flow of information. Yet fears of litigation stand as a major barrier to information flows and consequently are an indirect deterrent to establishing successful error reporting systems. Without protection from malpractice suits, how can health care professionals be willing to openly report error? Without an effective reporting system, how can reliable baseline data about errors be established?

The frustrating answer is that a focus on error reporting may be the wrong way to proceed. Studdert, Brennan, and Thomas make a sensible suggestion that the United States adopt a version of the Swedish no-fault insurance scheme for more equitable compensation. They even demonstrate that it would not cost any more and could even cost less than our current tort approach. However, as they recognize, it is highly unlikely that the United States will give up its tort system; the costs in terms of political will and determination are perhaps too great. Without a deep crisis in medical malpractice premiums, the will won't be there. Where does that leave us in developing useful reporting systems? Essentially stymied.

The key lessons from Studdert and his colleagues are that large empirical studies based on archival record reviews present enormous challenges and that the threat of litigation will undermine the comprehensiveness of mandatory and voluntary reporting systems. Consider, for example, that Sweden has had a mandatory reporting law (Lex Maria) since the 1930s for what we now call *sentinel events*. The reporting has been sparse to say the least, and this in a society that eschews the courts for settling such disputes (Rosenthal, 1987).

Although large empirical studies garner great attention, they are not the only source of data on medical errors and adverse events. Many small studies have been conducted over the last six decades, mostly by physicians (see Rosenthal, 1995, chap. 6), and reviews of a wide range of AE literature have been published in professional journals during the last four decades, in both the United States and Great Britain. These reviews address, for example, autopsy studies, studies of residents and fatigue, studies of maternal and infant deaths, and the famous British confidential inquiries into postoperative morbidity and mortality. The IOM report includes several of these reviews, including a separate review of prescription errors.

Although the research literature is extensive, it is still flawed in the sense that most studies use data gathered from medical records, which are often not only incomplete but also not used to report many AEs. Methodologies vary and definitions vary, as do interpretations and remedies. Meta-analysis of multiple studies would be useful. But it is not clear that additional large empirical studies would be worth the time and money they would take. It is likely that other approaches, some mentioned here in other chapters (see Chapter Eleven, for example), will produce better and more effective results in identifying, reducing, and preventing adverse events, mistakes, errors, and mishaps. We need to clarify our terminology and identify alternate approaches and think about other types of reporting systems. Strong clues to how this may be done are to be found in an analysis of the chapters in Parts Two and Three of this book.

Multiple Perspectives and Multiple Endeavors

At the heart of this volume are the perspectives of clinicians, administrators, and organizational scholars who share their views on
mistakes, how they are caused, and how they can be mitigated. This
section summarizes the key findings from these chapters and begins
to assess how various health care players think about medical
mishaps. Moreover, there are a large number of efforts already in
place that are attempting to improve care, many of which reach toward patient safety (see Appendix Two).

Darrell Campbell, a highly respected transplant surgeon and
medical leader, and his colleague Patricia Cornett take a bold, comprehensive look in Chapter Two at the relationships between stress
and burnout and medical mistakes. They review literature usually
out of the purview of surgeons. "The conclusion," they assert,
"seems inescapable that there is a strong association between high
levels of stress and burnout among health care workers and their
organizations and an increased propensity to commit medical mistakes of all kinds." At the same time, they acknowledge that even
though existing evidence is indirect and there is a need for studies
that directly and systematically investigate this association, there
is also an immediate need for practical steps to reduce potential
stressors. Although research linking stress and burnout with job
performance is extensive, medical culture presents many barriers to
concerted stress reduction efforts. Performance under stress is too
often perceived as a test of dedication and commitment, particularly in surgery, and as an important element in the socialization
and training of physicians.

Michael Fetters, a professor of family medicine, acknowledges
in Chapter Three that although the IOM report is focused mostly
on errors in inpatient settings and neglects errors in primary care
practice, its insistence on action must be applied to outpatient care
as well. As Fetters notes, primary care is both the primary portal of
entry into the U.S. health care system and the setting in which the

vast majority of patients receive care. Yet little empirical research is available on mishaps in outpatient settings.

Fetters suggests that the lack of convincing data on error prevalence is often construed as evidence that the primary care system is safe, and it may inadvertently contribute to complacence about both furthering research on errors in primary care and promoting action to make primary care safer. He discusses the barriers to building appropriate patient safety systems in office settings, including the requirements for time, resources, and financial incentives that currently do not exist. He calls for special continuing medical education modules, taxonomies relevant to primary care, and adaptation of the IOM's hospital-oriented suggestions. Finally, he raises questions about the applicability of systems safety models from the airline industry to outpatient care, noting, in particular, that it would be difficult to develop the standard operating routines and team collaboration these systems rely on given the wide variation in the types of medical problems seen on a typical day and in the structure and design of primary practice settings. Fetters remains hopeful, but the challenges and barriers he points out are formidable.

In Chapter Four, a chief of nursing, Beverly Jones, explores with considerable sensitivity the culture of medical practice that physicians and nurses share. She laments its emphasis, for both nurses and doctors, on aiming for personal perfection and on the "code of silence" that has dominated the way these professionals have dealt with error. She also finds that systems analysis offers considerable hope for discovering how the organization of work that surrounds clinical practice contributes to individual mistakes. She worries about the way that the deeply entrenched, quiet agreement not to discuss mistakes outside the tight circles of practitioners will prevent the useful and more open disclosure needed to improve patient safety. She emphasizes the conflict between clinical autonomy and effective monitoring and notes how shared experiences of mistakes often make collegial criticism difficult. She also laments the hierarchy of relationships in hospitals that suppresses contributions from all members of the clinical team. For nurses the environment is one of "passivity and silence." It is this chapter that points to the sources of the major professional barriers to mishap detection, examination, reduction, and prevention.

Michael Millenson's "The Patient's View of Medical Errors" (Chapter Five) is a powerful and painful picture of how individual patient experiences, rendered in journalistic style, reflect and shape mass perception and action. From one perspective, the patient point of view is a perfect reflection of much that can be criticized about the mass media. From another perspective, this chapter reflects the one hundred–year history of events that has brought medical errors out into the open. From the former perspective, the chapter reflects black-and-white caricatures where patients are always exploited and doctors are always negligent. There is a sensationalizing of the mistakes; journalists are characterized as saviors; the IOM report is beyond criticism. The courts are the best avenues of redress, systems concepts from the airline industry will be the saviors of the hospitals, and an anecdote makes a trend.

Hospitals are chastised for letting incompetent doctors remain on staff, but the hundreds of hospitals unable to withdraw privileges because of counter lawsuits are never mentioned. The chapter clearly reflects the time and space limitations of most forms of journalism and the enormous pressure the media are under to sell papers, expand audiences, and increase advertising.

From the latter perspective, however, this chapter chronicles the evolving role of the patient from passive observer in the doctor-patient relationship to active participant in that relationship. Increasing patient activism is often attributed to recent advances in information technology and the increased availability of relevant information. Yet the call for patient safety has probably also fostered patient involvement in self-care by increasing the likelihood that doctors will be more proactive in acknowledging and communicating medical uncertainties and risks (Pichert & Hickson, 2001).

Careful and accurate journalism has an important role to play in informing the public and encouraging intelligent public discussion. This chapter underscores the absolutely vital task of educating the media and the public with accurate, reliable, and nonsensational information. But, perversely, it also reminds us that it often takes sensation to create a strong enough force for change. Perhaps what will save us from the irresponsibility of many in the media will be responsibly administered Web pages easily accessible to the public. Then determined patients will have ready access to better sources of information. But they will have to learn how to identify the reliable and ignore the nonsense that sullies the medium of the Web too. And there will still be those who are unable to get accurate information and who will then depend on the least reliable media sources.

Trying to Manage Error: What We Do Now

It is amazing how many quality assurance efforts are currently swarming among the various layers of health care. Appendixes One and Two illustrate that health care professionals and organizations have hardly ignored problems of quality and error. The number of activities is substantial and the pace is frenetic. Voluntary and regulatory pressures from external sources drive some of this activity. Bodenheimer (1999) lists all the organizations able to negotiate hospitals and doctors into continuous quality improvement efforts: the National Committee for Quality Assurance (NCQA) with the Health Plan Employer Data and Information Set (HEDIS), the Joint Commission on Accreditation of Healthcare Organizations (JCAHO) with ORYX®, the CMS with the Quality Improvement System for Managed Care (QISMC), the Institute for Health Care Improvement, the Agency for Healthcare Research and Quality (AHRQ), the National Patient Safety Foundation (NPSF), the National Roundtable on Health Care Quality, the Consumer Coalition, the Leapfrog Group, and the recent six sigma challenge (Chassin, 1998).

Bodenheimer concludes by noting market-driven health care will work toward quality only if it is "rewarded in the market for doing so" (p. 492).

In addition to the extensive catalogue of academic medical centers' continuous quality assurance efforts, Part Three of this book examines three particular contexts for error reduction: administrative protocols in managed care organizations, administrative risk management departments of hospitals, and physician-led work in evidence-based medicine and outcomes research. The extent and depth of the efforts in these contexts is impressive. However, they need to be scrutinized with three questions in mind: What have they contributed to error reduction? Why haven't they contributed more? Why haven't their contributions been more widely recognized?

One important response can be found in Beverly Jones's chapter, "Nurses and the 'Code of Silence.'" This answer has much to do with the medical profession's deep training for and commitment to autonomy, self-regulation, and knowledge monopoly and all that accrues from these essential characteristics, particularly suspicion and distrust of administrative incursions into medical territory. More discussion of this important observation will be presented later in this chapter.

Derek van Amerongen has deep faith in the quality assurance systems that a managed care organization (MCO) can mount and their ability to substantially reduce error, and in Chapter Six, he recounts Anthem Blue Cross Blue Shield's efforts to do so. Consistent data collection, physician profiling and feedback, promotion of evidence-based medicine, and converting outcomes research into practice guidelines all show great promise, he claims. It is too soon to determine whether these efforts will make good on their promises because little evidence has yet accumulated on the specific causal processes that support these claims. An important implication of van Amerongen's perspective is that an MCO can provide useful feedback from which doctors and other health care providers can learn.

Susan Horn, Joanne Hickey, Theresa Carroll, and Anne-Claire France make the same case, in rich detail, for evidence-based medicine and the clinical practice improvement (CPI) methodology that is gaining popularity among clinicians as an important means of discovering best treatments and processes for specified patient types. In Chapter Eight, Horn and her colleagues make a compelling case for the advantages of CPI over randomized controlled trials, even though it is too early to empirically substantiate the benefits of CPI. An important implication of CPI is that the process may be robust enough to lead to effective and safe practices that can be broadly applied to a variety of everyday medical treatments and in a variety of medical settings. The challenge is to avoid cookie-cutter approaches.

Margaret Dawson, Ann Munro, Kenneth Appleby, and Susan Anderson, in "Risk Management and Medical Errors" (Chapter Seven), make an elaborate case that risk management departments, units that exist in almost every hospital in the United States, are currently trying to reshape themselves to assist their hospitals to respond to the public demands and pressure aroused by the IOM report. Risk management has a history to overcome first. Its roots lie in predicting and conserving *risk loss* in terms of financial health, possible litigation, and harm to reputation, rather than in facilitating *safety*. The well-known incident reports rarely include incidents in which doctors are involved but seem to focus on nurses and other allied health professionals. Although risk managers certainly have the potential to contribute to reducing medical mistakes in everyday situations, particularly by identifying error trends and raising specific issues for further study and analysis, they have a long way to go before they enter the heart of clinical practice and are trusted by the profession of medicine. As the IOM report notes (Kohn et al., 2000, p. 221), "risk management has not been embraced at the organizational leadership level" nor, one may add, with any enthusiasm by clinicians for other than nonphysician incidents.

A theme common to all three chapters is the resistance of physicians to proposed bureaucratic interventions. Such resistance has of course long been a topic in organizational behavior literature, which is replete with discussion, studies, and theories about the conflict between professional culture and organizational culture. Scott (1984, 1987), one of the distinguished scholars of this clash, has written since the 1960s about the conflict between managers and physicians in hospitals. He noted in his 1984 paper that as organizations like hospitals become more complex, managers more professionalized, and external environments more demanding, conflicts would increase. Increasingly emboldened managers, administrators, and bureaucrats, both inside and outside health care systems and hospitals, have increasingly challenged the intrinsic characteristics of medical professional culture, particularly those that surround the cherished value of autonomy (Freidson, 1970; Goode, 1957). The profession of medicine has powerful tools with which to resist managerial incursions such as quality assurance initiatives that approach the prerogatives of clinical autonomy. These tools include the profession's knowledge monopoly and its role as patient advocate (Rosenthal, 1999). Yet it is important also to note that doctors' need to exercise discretion in some critical areas of their work is not necessarily inconsistent with the precise specification of other aspects of their performance. In other words, standard procedures and specifications may be inappropriate for some highly complex and uncertain tasks (for example, a particular surgery) yet very appropriate for other tasks (for example, providing certain information in every patient handoff).

Systems Theories: Are They Applicable?

Are systems theories and models for understanding and reducing error appropriate and useful to error reduction in medicine? Part Four of this book provides unique insights and answers to this question.

In Chapter Nine, Karl Weick, a renowned social psychologist, says yes, but only if leaders in health care understand systems theories correctly. He is deeply disturbed at the misinterpretation and misrepresentation of systems and systems theories in the IOM report and by the medical leaders who have been strongly touting systems theories and models for error detection and reduction from industry, particularly the aviation industry. He laments the distorted focus on system as a static, mechanical, routinized entity and highlights the point that current theories drastically underestimate the dynamic features, such as unfolding events and the role of interdependencies, in the generation of adverse medical events. He eloquently explains that relationships, organizational culture, and a number of processes contribute to collective *mindfulness* and that all these must be better understood—and changed—if errors are to be caught and corrected before disastrous results occur.

Paul Schulman, also a distinguished systems theorist, takes a different view in Chapter Ten. Systems theories and models developed for corporate and industrial organizations may not be wholly relevant to the world of clinical medicine and medical mistakes. He asks, in his title, "How Reliable Is Reliability Theory?" referring to the theory with which he (and Weick) is closely identified and the process of turning high risk organizations into high reliability organizations. His answer is let us be very, very cautious.

Schulman deplores the generalization that medical error is like error in any other industry. He wisely calls for an understanding that error is not only different in medicine as a whole but that it can mean very different things in different specialties. This is a striking suggestion, as is his admonition not to think we can import wholesale reliability strategies from other industries. We should welcome this crucial caution, along with Schulman's assertion that important improvements can be made in medical procedures, training, and supervision.

Schulman also devotes considerable space to pointing out the high levels of achievement already accomplished in medicine. This stands in refreshing contrast to the IOM report's absurd accusations (echoed in Chapter Five) about disinterest and neglect in the medical profession and hospitals. The IOM report would have been considerably strengthened in its realistic usefulness had it suggested cautions and reserve in regard to systems applications, rather than attempting to drive medical care willy-nilly into the wholesale embrace of industrial safety models.

Finally, Chapter Eleven discusses a responsible attempt to apply models for detection and prevention from the airline industry to the hospital operating room. Eric Thomas (a physician) and Robert Helmreich (an industrial organizational psychologist) point out what they consider to be the similarities and the differences between the pilot and the surgeon and anesthesiologist and between the airline cockpit and the hospital operating room.

The differences are myriad. But Thomas and Helmreich see enough similarities to attempt to adapt various airline safety systems to the operating room. They provide a picture of the various techniques used by the airline industry to collect error data (surveys, protected incident reports, and direct observation) and of the simulation and crew resource management used to improve team alertness to safety. Their initial findings are well worth our close examination.

In surveys comparing the attitudes of pilots and medical personnel toward the effects of fatigue, hierarchical teams, and the appropriateness of acknowledging and discussing errors, the medical personnel come out on the short side in each category, meaning that they typically underestimate the importance of these factors. Thomas and Helmreich find medical incident reporting relatively immature and not well evaluated compared to reporting in the airline industry. And they find little evidence of the effectiveness of mandatory and voluntary reporting systems in medicine. The use of direct observation in the operating room reveals that setting to be more complex than the cockpit; individual patients are less predictable than airplanes; teamwork and communications are often suboptimal compared to cockpit behavior. Crew resource management techniques from the airline industry must be applied with caution and only after understanding the culture of the operating room. Thomas and Helmreich conclude that the usefulness of aviation models in reducing medical error and improving patient safety is promising but far from proven. And they urge caution, so as to avoid blindly adopting the aviation approach without establishing its validity through solid research.

Perhaps this book's greatest contribution to improving patient safety will be this section on systems theories, a judicious and informed collection of discussions from systems thinkers and a team of researchers in the forefront of efforts to apply industry safety models to error reduction and improved patient safety in medicine.

Indeed, other cautionary tales are emerging about attempted applications of industry models to health care. The big auto manufacturers have been offering their hospital and health system contractors the services of the quality improvement teams they have been sending to their industrial contractors. One quality improvement team plan for redesigning an emergency department resulted in a 70 percent staff attrition rate, followed by a rapid drift back to the department's original organization (Rosenthal, 2001). The auto industry team members came away from that experience recognizing they had failed and admitting to having "learned a great deal."

Here are the best reasons for proceeding cautiously and carefully. Certainly we must have serious study of the safety experiences from other organizational sectors of society, but at the same time we must identify what is necessarily unique in medical care and medical culture. Caution and thoughtfulness are difficult to accomplish in an atmosphere politicized with calls for immediate action. Nevertheless, immediate action is often ill-informed action and usually provides solutions that are themselves the source of new errors and new problems.

Understanding and Engaging the Profession of Medicine

The weight of this book leads in one clear direction. It points to the overwhelming need to understand the culture of medicine, medicine's unique body of knowledge, the way the profession views its work, and the intrinsic, shifting uncertainties that surround the care that clinical services offer. Without an understanding that uncertainty lies in the deep heart of medicine (Fox, 1957/1969; Rosenthal, 1999) and without an understanding of the ways uncertainty shapes medical culture, outside efforts to promote patient safety will produce only short-lived results, if that.

Renee Fox's landmark 1957 study explored the various forms of uncertainty in clinical medicine. Charles Bosk published a now classic study, *Forgive and Remember: Managing Medical Failure* (1979), that documents the emphasis doctors place on the process of clinical work in the face of medical uncertainty. And Rosenthal (1995), in exploring the informal techniques doctors use when dealing with colleagues who are the source of problems, found that medical uncertainty figured prominently in how doctors think about their work. What is evident from these studies is that uncertainty has influenced the evolution of professional medical culture.

Sociologists of medicine usually accept Freidson's characterization of the medical profession, which includes the following elements: high ethical and service orientations; a selection and educational process that is rigorous, demanding, and professionally controlled; and training and socialization processes that are particularly comprehensive and that produce strong individual identification with the profession as a whole and control through self-regulation and autonomy (clinical, economic, and political). These elements arose in the profession precisely because the nature of doctors' work is uncertain and complex. But these same elements of the profession periodically come under attack. And this stage in the development of the U.S. health care system has come at just such a period (see Rosenthal, 1987, for a discussion of waxing and waning autonomy).

A recurring theme in these and other studies is that uncertainty undergirds the way doctors think about their work and about adverse events. Without an understanding of the stark realities of medical uncertainty, the culture that has grown from it, and the fierce loyalty most doctors have to that culture, little progress will be made in improving patient safety.

On the one hand, one implication of these studies is that the medical profession must lead and dominate all patient safety efforts if such efforts are to be successful. Doctors need to make these efforts their own. This is not a difficult goal. The overwhelming majority of doctors want to help their patients. Who can believe otherwise? They do need to be supported and, yes, prodded from the outside. Medical leaders will have a hard task in moving the middle mass of the profession because of the characteristics of the profession and because it is always difficult to change entrenched ways of behaving. Social pressure seems necessary; the IOM report is a powerful pressure. But if the profession does not engage in these efforts on its own terms, they will not be carried out. Those who have a knowledge and skills monopoly and are closest to patients have continuing power even when under attack. Although the allied health professions have broadened the bounds of their legitimate domains of expertise and responsibility, the knowledge authority of the medical profession has been little changed by its competitors.

On the other hand, to suggest that physicians take the lead or work independently on these matters may be problematic. It is well known that individuals are subject to numerous cognitive biases and develop worldviews that are based both on their experience and their position in an organizational structure. So it is not surprising that multiple perspectives are crucial in the construction and perceptions of problems and their solutions.

Karl Weick (see Chapter Nine) recounts the idea that experts often overestimate their likelihood of recognizing a phenomenon if it were actually taking place. This *fallacy of centrality*—"if I don't know about this event, it must not be happening"—is seriously damaging, because it discourages curiosity on the part of the person adopting it and also "frequently creates in him/her an antagonistic stance toward the events in question" (Weick, 1995, p. 2). In addition, Weick notes that people tend to see what they are able to deal with. The backlash and resistance to public pressures for patient safety may arise in part from professional culture, but one might also argue that part of the resistance is physicians' inability to believe that their own evaluation of the dangerousness of medical care could be seriously in error or that they might not know what to do about it.

The results we all want will come when we cooperate to find the most effective ways of understanding and managing these uncertain and complex situations. If the various interest groups sense that their situations are respected, they will respect and seek insights from other fields and disciplines. We can begin by attempting to understand the unique ways doctors talk about their work. The very language of error within the profession reveals a great deal about the subjective side of medical care and the complexities of the health care system. And it also reveals that we are not all talking about the same thing when we talk about patient safety.

Sorting Out the Terminology; Recognizing Complexity and Uncertainty

Adverse event, anticipated and *unanticipated consequence, mistake, error, preventable adverse event, negligent adverse event, potential adverse event* (that is, a *near miss*)—all these terms, and more, are found in discussions of what we now have accepted as a common umbrella term and useful euphemism, *patient safety*. *Safety* may be defined as freedom from accidental injury. The term *patient safety* recognizes that this is the primary safety goal from the patient's perspective. The term *patient safety* itself is a recent, masterful choice of terminology, making discussion more acceptable to the medical profession and the public at large. It has a positive meaning and, rather than pointing the finger of blame at doctors, puts the emphasis on improving care for patients through the establishment of operational systems and processes that minimize the likelihood of errors and maximize the likelihood of intercepting errors when they are about to occur (Kohn et al., 2000).

Many Words, Many Meanings

Vocabulary can be a powerful source of confusion in communication. We may share a common language, but that is never a guarantee that we understand each other. The terminology with which medical mistakes are discussed is a perfect example of likely confusion.

The terms used to describe errors and adverse events in the medical literature can be grouped into two broad categories (Vincent, 2001). Terms such as *error, mishap,* and *mistake* usually describe a deviation in processes of care, which may or may not cause harm to patients. The word *mistake,* according to *Merriam-Webster's Collegiate Dictionary* (9th ed.), means "a wrong action proceeding from faulty judgment, inadequate knowledge, or inattention," and this meaning is likely to be consistent with what a patient is thinking of when referring to a medical mistake. Terms such as *adverse event* refer to undesired patient outcomes that may or may not be the result of errors. Adverse events may be anticipated or unanticipated. A *preventable adverse event* occurs when an injury results from substandard medical care and is likely to be consistent with what the legal system conceives of as an error or mistake. When a jury finds against a doctor or a hospital, the popular perception is that of *negligence,* the "failure to exercise the care that a prudent person usually exercises" (*Merriam-Webster's Collegiate Dictionary*); the doctor was careless, ignorant, lacking in skills. (For a complete discussion of terms and definitions see Appendix One).

The meaning of a term may be shaped by the context in which the people who are using that term are situated. For the medical profession, the meaning of *mistake* is shaped by a work context of uncertainty. For the legal system, it is defined in the context of a predetermined set of rules and definitions laid out in legal codes and legal thinking. For the public, it is defined in the context of what seems to have gone wrong relative to a set of preconceived and highly individualized expectations.

Communicating in a Context of Uncertainty

Doctors and other health professionals routinely communicate uncertainty and risks to patients and their families, but they do this through the lens of the uncertainty they understand. For example, a doctor may inform the patient about his or her condition, the treatment, the prognosis, significant complications, risks, benefits, alternative treatments available, and any additional information required that may be necessary to give informed consent prior to a procedure. But this ideal is rarely achieved in daily practice because doctors face a number of challenges in communicating all the uncertainties that are part of the information. These challenges revolve around the difficulties of identifying the risks themselves, because they may not be completely known or understood; of conveying risk probabilities; of choosing which risks to discuss; and of accurately discerning the extent to which a patient wants to be involved in decision making and at what level of understanding (Pichert & Hickson, 2001). And there is no single standard for making these determinations. Moreover, research suggests that many other obstacles are associated with risk communication. What is important here is that these challenges embody many of the elements of uncertainty that doctors gradually learn to live with beginning in medical school, then in residency training, and finally in independent practice (Fox, 1957/1969; Bosk, 1979).

At the same time that they are called on to be authoritative, doctors must also accept the intrinsic uncertainty of their work (Rosenthal, 1997). Furthermore there is convincing evidence that the reality of uncertainty shapes not only the way they think about their work but how they think about mistakes in particular.

Although the shape and size of uncertainty varies from specialty to specialty, patient to patient, and situation to situation, its presence is the one certainty of the practice of medicine (Paget, 1988).

The voices of the practitioners in Part Two of this book show distinct traces of this thinking. For example, Campbell and Cornett write in Chapter Two, "Uncertainty about outcomes is at the core of modern medical practice. . . . [S]ome of the factors surrounding uncertainty in medical decision making [are] ambiguity of relevant data, lack of understanding of basic biological processes, and the need to act before all information can be gathered."

Doctors need to be authoritative. That is how they are taught to behave, and some patients want that authoritativeness because it enhances their trust of the doctor and the treatments they may be subjected to. However, it is difficult to be authoritative and at the same time to convey the probabilistic nature of medicine and its uncertainty, an uncertainty that doctors themselves have long ago accepted. Moreover, it is also true that sometimes some doctors hide their own inadequacies behind claims that medicine is inherently uncertain. Some even claim there is no such thing as a medical mistake (Rosenthal, 1995). But of course there is. Medical mistakes are the product of individual factors such as a lack of knowledge, lack of experience and skill, temporary distractions, or impairment; they are the product of organizational and systems factors such as faulty communication, conflict, information overload, task ambiguity, conflicting goals, cognitive biases, awkward technology, or work environments that don't try (or are unable) to protect against resource or staffing shortages, stress, fatigue, and myriad other barriers to patient safety.

Shrinking the Borders of Uncertainty

Error identification in medicine is still in its infancy. And improving it will not be an easy process. The difficulties in error identification stem in part from the inherent uncertainty and subjectivity of medical care and in part from the complex nature of our health care systems. A *complex system* is one in which a change can have unpredictable effects. It is impossible to say unequivocally that any given action will have a positive effect, a negative effect, or no effect at all on this system. These factors complicate the search for solutions to this vexing issue of error identification. How can we distinguish when individual or systems inadequacies are the problem and when medical uncertainty is the problem? Fox brought this general question to health care professionals' attention in her 1957 study of medical students, where she described three uncertainties medical students (and we can safely say practicing physicians) face: (1) the uncertainties of their own knowledge and skills; (2) the uncertainties in medical knowledge; and (3) the uncertainty of how to distinguish between the two.

Herein lies the real challenge in discussing adverse events, medical errors, systems errors, and reduction and prevention, one that repeatedly shows up in discussions of medical mistakes and patient safety. It is the difficulty of distinguishing between errors and adverse events. We have highlighted that actions sometimes become errors only in retrospect. Actions that appear entirely reasonable at one point in time may at a later point in time be identified as errors when an adverse outcome ensues. Conversely actions recognized as errors may not result in an adverse outcome.

When we talk about mistakes in medicine and reducing them, we are talking about a particularly complex subject. No one solution will do; no one theory will suffice. We need to recognize different categories of mistakes and then proceed differentially and appropriately and without pressured haste.

We also need to push the members of the medical profession and challenge their thinking about *nonpreventable adverse events*. How many instances are there of better technology reducing known and accepted risks? A perfect example of this is the recent development of improved catheters that reduce catheter-related infections by a third to a half (Saint, Veentra, Sullivan, Chenoweth, & Fendrick, 2000). These infection rates never got into incident reports; they are not counted or mentioned in the literature on medical mistakes. For some time they have been accepted as a nonpreventable, acceptable risk of using catheters.

This example suggests that doctors would do well to review periodically all the "nonpreventable" adverse events they can think of related to their particular specialty. They could also examine what they and their specialty colleagues consider preventable adverse events and determine why they occur. How many of these can be addressed with improved technology? Improved technique? Faster transmission of bench research to the bedside? Less stress? This is a more fruitful (and positive) approach to detection, reduction, and prevention of adverse events than the use of reporting systems, counting, and large-scale studies.

We need to help the profession keep shrinking the borders of uncertainty, even as new technologies enter the field and create new uncertainties, and to encourage physicians to systematically and regularly challenge their own concepts of adverse events, particularly ones they have perceived as nonpreventable.

An Agenda for Future Action, Research, and Education

Taken together, the contributions to this volume suggest that there is much to be done. The following agenda offers some general recommendations for action, education, and research.

Action

- Encourage each specialty to identify areas in which patient safety can be improved, emphasizing preventable adverse events. Establish current baseline data; announce changes, implement changes, and evaluate improvement. Set realistic goals for realistic time periods. For example, in May 2000, the Society for Academic Emergency Medicine sponsored a conference on errors in emergency medicine to explore error, to develop a meaningful research agenda, and to stimulate systematic action and research in this area.

- Adopt information technology such as computer-based patient tracking systems and computerized order-entry and computer-assisted decision-making systems. Accumulating evidence suggests that these systems not only improve care but also are cost effective. Best practices need to be shared so late adopters can avoid pitfalls. Enact small changes whenever possible, and disseminate best practices. Change is difficult in every organization. Medical culture makes it even more difficult. Moreover, large-scale, top-down change programs rarely produce change. Start with small, focused projects that have a better chance of succeeding, and then disseminate the results widely.

- Use informal cultural norms. Create an error-friendly learning culture in which errors can be surfaced and learning can take place. Learning is curtailed when people in a position to initiate learning perceive they are placing their career or their image at risk if they admit an error, ask for help, or seek feedback. Through actions and expectations, create a climate of openness in which people feel it is safe to surface unexpected events rather than covering them up, ask for help if they need it, and seek feedback. Make it easy for people to confess errors. Although learning mechanisms such as morbidity and mortality conferences have traditionally been a primary mechanism for learning, research shows that for feedback to be effective it must be provided as quickly as possible after an event. A culture in which people can surface errors and get prompt and helpful feedback is a culture in which learning is more likely to take place.

- Involve residents in developing a priority list of action items for error reduction. Newcomers in a system may raise naïve questions that lead to new ways to make a system better. Teach residents techniques to handle stress and offer mental health support programs.

- Consider making the previous actions part of hospital accreditation requirements.

- Form interdisciplinary teams that include people with expertise in the safety sciences (those knowledgeable in reliability theory, organizational behavior and change, cognitive psychology, anthropology, sociology, or human factors engineering, for example) along with physicians, nurses, pharmacists, and so forth, to tackle problems.

Research

- Evaluate the effectiveness of interventions aimed at enhancing performance and mitigating adverse outcomes. For example, at appropriate intervals, examine an effort to reduce adverse drug events by initiating information systems for direct order entry.

- Target high-incidence areas for studies of preventable adverse events. Although the exact rate of preventable adverse events in medicine is not known, it is suspected that the incidence in some areas, such as the emergency department, is possibly orders of magnitude higher than in other areas. Start in these suspect areas.

- Evaluate a variety of research paradigms, and triangulate by using multiple research traditions. The epidemiological model may be familiar to many physicians, but it is not clear that this model is or will be the most successful. Use multiple methods, including observational studies, to achieve a richer understanding of the complex environment in which adverse events occur.

- Evaluate the efficacy of physician profiling in changing physician behavior. The characteristics profiled should be controlled by physicians and privately reviewed within specialty groups.

Education

- Include the topics of patient safety and medical error in medical school curricula. Discuss patient safety and medical error explicitly; provide students with specific examples. Encourage teams of residents to form study groups on adverse events they see in practice. Promote continuing medical education (CME) courses.

- Educate the public more broadly about medical uncertainty, medical error, and the incidence of error. Highlight that uncovering error is the first step to preventing error and that the existence of error in a health care facility does not necessarily mean that the institution is dangerous or that the physicians are bad.

Conclusion

Many people, prodded by the newspapers and politicians, want immediate action. Such rapid action usually leads to hastily thought out and quickly implemented programs that do not have much chance to work. Of course we need action! However, we need thoughtful action based on the best research or sustained clinical experience possible.

People often have a strong temptation to simplify. Everything then looks easy. Yet changing large, complex systems and their practices is seldom easy, and we always pay a price in the long run when we trust simple descriptions, answers, and solutions.

These are exciting and challenging times. They offer opportunities that demand creativity, innovation, and new thinking — tremendous opportunities. But they require clear struggles as well: a struggle to open our minds to other disciplines and understand what they might have to offer that we can adapt, a struggle to act thoughtfully by understanding and overcoming cultural and organizational barriers to change.

It is time to grasp these exciting opportunities and engage in these struggles so the health care profession can renew and reclaim its role in serving patients.

References

Andrews, L. B., Stocking, C., Krizek, T., Gottlieb, L., Krizek, C., Vargish, T., & Siegler, M. (1997, February 1). An alternative strategy for studying adverse events in medical care. *Lancet, 349,* 309–313.

Bodenheimer, T. (1999, February 11). The American health care system: The movement for improved quality in health care. *New England Journal of Medicine, 340,* 488–492.

Bosk, C. (1979). *Forgive and remember: Managing medical failure.* Chicago: University of Chicago Press.

Brennan, T. A., Leape, L. L., Laird, N. M., Herbert, L. E., Localio, A. R., Lawthers, A. G., Newhouse, J. P., Weiler, P. C., & Hiatt, H. H. (1991). Incidence of adverse events and negligence in hospitalized patients: Results of the Harvard Medical Practice Study I. *New England Journal of Medicine, 324,* 370–376.

Chassin, M. R. (1998). Is health care ready for six sigma quality? *Milbank Memorial Quarterly, 76*(4), 565–591.

Committee on Quality of Health Care in America, Institute of Medicine. (2001). *Crossing the quality chasm: A new health system for the 21st century.* Washington, DC: National Academy Press.

Fox, R. (1957/1969). Training for uncertainty. In R. Merton, G. Reader, & P. Kendall (Eds.), *The student physician* (pp. 207–241). Cambridge: Harvard University Press.

Freidson, E. (1970). *The profession of medicine: A study of the sociology of applied knowledge.* New York: HarperCollins.

Goode, W. (1957). Community within a community: The professions. *American Sociological Review, 25,* 902–914.

Kohn, L. T., Corrigan, J. M., & Donaldson, M. S. (Eds.); Committee on Quality of Health Care in America, Institute of Medicine. (2000). *To err is human: Building a safer health system*. Washington, DC: National Academy Press.

Mills, D. H. (1978, April). Medical Insurance Feasibility Study: A technical summary. *Western Journal of Medicine, 128*, 360–365.

Paget, M. (1988). *The unity of mistakes: A phenomenological interpretation of medical work*. Philadelphia: Temple University Press.

Pichert, J. W., & Hickson, G. B. (2001). Communicating risks to patients and families. In C. Vincent (Ed.), *Clinical risk management: Enhancing patient safety* (2nd ed., pp. 263–282). London: BMJ Books.

Rosenthal, M. M. (1987). *Dealing with medical malpractice: The British and Swedish experience*. London: Tavistock.

Rosenthal, M. M. (1995). *The incompetent doctor: Behind closed doors*. Bristol, PA: Open University Press.

Rosenthal, M. M. (1997). Knowledge monopoly, uncertainty and regulation of the medical profession. *British Medical Journal, 314*, 1633.

Rosenthal, M. M. (1999). Medical uncertainty, medical collegiality and improving quality of care. In J. Kronenfield (Ed.), *Sociological research* (Vol. 16, pp. 3–30). Greenwich, CT: JAI Press.

Rosenthal, M. M. (2001, January). Unpublished interview with an emergency department director.

Saint, S., Veentra, D. L., Sullivan, S. D., Chenoweth, C., & Fendrick, A. M. (2000). The potential clinical and economic benefits of silver alloy urinary catheters in preventing urinary tract infection. *Archives of Internal Medicine, 160*, 2670–2675.

Scott, W. R. (1984, May 4–5). *Conflicting levels of rationality: Regulators, managers and professionals in the medical setting*. Lecture delivered at the Graduate Program in Health Administration, University of Chicago.

Scott, W. R. (1987). *Organizations: Rational, natural, and open systems*. Upper Saddle River, NJ: Prentice Hall.

Thomas, E. J., Studdert, D. M., Burstin, H. R., Orav, J., Zeena, T., Williams, E. J., Howard, K. M., Weiler, P. C., & Brennan, T. A. (2000). Incidence and types of adverse events and negligent care in Utah and Colorado. *Medical Care, 38*, 261–271.

Vincent, C. (2001). *Clinical risk management: Enhancing patient safety* (2nd ed.). London: BMJ Books.

Weick, K. E. (1995). *Sensemaking in organizations*. Thousand Oaks, CA: Sage.

Wilson, R. M., Runciman, W. B., Gibberd, R. W., Harrison, B. T., Newby, L., and Hamilton, J. D. (1995, November 6). The Quality in Australian Health Care Study. *Medical Journal of Australia, 163*, 458–471.

Appendix One

A Collection of Definitions

Adam Scheffler, Lorri Zipperer, and Susan Cushman

What These Definitions Are— and What They Are Not

[For this glossary] we have selected terms that represent major concepts important to the discussion of patient safety. . . . We do not intend this collection to be exhaustive, "official," or determinative in a legal or policy sense. Researchers, practitioners, legislators, regulators, and accrediting agencies all continue to debate the meanings of several fundamental terms in use, such as "error," "mistake," and "safety." We encourage readers who wish to follow these debates to seek out relevant books, reports, journal articles, news coverage, workshops, conferences, and on-line forums.

Accident

An unplanned, unexpected, and undesired event, usually with an adverse consequence.

Senders JW.
Medical devices, medical errors, and medical accidents.

Appendix One is reprinted from *Lessons in Patient Safety*, edited by Lorri Zipperer and Susan Wagner Cushman, published by the National Patient Safety Foundation 2001. Used by permission. *Lessons in Patient Safety* is available from the National Patient Safety Foundation, 515 North State Street, Chicago, IL 60610; tel. 312-464-4848, or via its Web site at www.npsf.org.

In: Bogner MS, ed.
Human Error in Medicine.
Hillsdale, NJ: Lawrence Erlbaum Associates. 1994. [166]

Active failures

Errors and violations committed at the "sharp end" of the system —
by pilots, air traffic controllers, police officers, insurance brokers,
financial traders, ships' crews, control room operators, maintenance
personnel, and the like. Such unsafe acts are likely to have a direct
impact on the safety of the system and, because of the immediacy
of their adverse effects, these acts are termed *active* failures.

Reason J.
Managing the Risks of Organizational Accidents.
Aldershot, UK: Ashgate. 1997. [10]

Adverse drug event (ADE)

An injury resulting from medical intervention related to a drug.

Bates DW, Spell N, Cullen DJ, et al.
The costs of adverse drug events in hospitalized patients.
JAMA. 1997;277:307–311. [308]

Adverse event

An injury that was caused by medical management (rather than underlying disease) and that prolonged the hospitalization, produced
a disability at the time of discharge, or both.

Brennan TA, Leape LL, Laird NM, et al.
Incidence of adverse events and negligence in hospitalized patients.
Results of the Harvard Medical Practice Study I.
N Engl J Med. 1991;324:370–376. [370]

Benign errors

Events which cause no harm or lack an adverse outcome. Also referred to as "precursor events" or "near misses."

Battles JB, Kaplan HS, Van der Schaaf TW, Shea CE.
The attributes of medical event—reporting systems: experience
with a prototype medical event—reporting system for transfusion
medicine.
Arch Pathol Lab Med. 1998;122:231–238. [232]

Blunt end

[W]here regulatory, administrative, and organizational factors reside. . . . The blunt end of the system is the source of the resources
and constraints that form the environment where practitioners
work. The blunt end is also the source of demands for production
that sharp end practitioners must meet.

Cook RI, Woods DD, Miller C.
A Tale of Two Stories. Contrasting Views of Patient Safety.
Chicago: National Patient Safety Foundation. 1998. [13]
Available at: www.npsf.org/exec/report.html.

Cognitive science

An amalgamation of disciplines including artificial intelligence,
neuroscience, philosophy, and psychology. Within cognitive science, cognitive psychology is an umbrella discipline for those interested in cognitive activities such as perception, learning, memory,
language, concept formation, problem solving, and thinking.

Bogner MS.
Introduction.
In: Bogner MS, ed.
Human Error in Medicine.
Hillsdale, NJ: Lawrence Erlbaum Associates. 1994. [6]

Critical incident

A human error or equipment failure that could have led (if not discovered or corrected in time) or did lead to an undesirable outcome,
ranging from increased length of hospital stay to death.

Cooper JB, Newbower RS, Kitz, RJ.
An analysis of major errors and equipment failures in anesthesia management: considerations for prevention and detection.
Anesthesiology. 1984;60:34–42. [35]

Critical incident technique

A set of procedures for collecting direct observations of human behavior in such a way as to facilitate their potential usefulness in solving practical problems and developing broad psychological principles.

Flanagan JC.
The critical incident technique.
Psychol Bull. 1954;51:327–358. [327]

Error

The failure of a planned action to be completed as intended or use of a wrong plan to achieve an aim; the accumulation of errors results in accidents.

Kohn LT, Corrigan JM, Donaldson MS, eds.
To Err Is Human: Building a Safer Health System.
Washington, DC: National Academy Press. 2000. [210]
Available at: http://books.nap.edu/html/to_err_is_human.

Error in judgment/error of negligence

Often, a distinction can be made between error in judgment (ie, error simply related to flawed reasoning) and error of negligence (ie, error due to inattention or lack of obligatory effort).

Couch, NP, Tilney NL, Rayner AA, Moore FD.
The high cost of low-frequency events: The anatomy and economics of surgical mishaps.
N Engl J Med. 1981;304:634–637. [637]

Failure mode effect and criticality analysis

The systematic assessment of a process or product that enables one to determine the location and mechanism of potential failures.

Williams E, Talley R.
The use of failure mode effect and criticality analysis in a medication error subcommittee.
Hosp Pharm. 1994;29:331–332,334–336,339. [331]

Five Rights of Medication Administration

Right patient, right drug, right dose, right time, and right route.

Wakefield DS, Wakefield BJ, Borders T, Uden-Holman T, Blegen M, Vaughn T.
Understanding and comparing differences in reported medication administration error rates.
Am J Medical Qual. 1999;14(2):73–80. [74]

Fixation error

The *persistent* failure to revise a diagnosis or plan in the face of readily available evidence that suggests a revision is necessary.

Gaba DM.
Human error in dynamic medical domains.
In: Bogner MS, ed.
Human Error in Medicine.
Hillsdale, NJ: Lawrence Erlbaum Associates. 1994. [217]

Genotype of an incident

The characteristic collection of factors that lead to the surface, phenotypical appearance of the event. Genotypes refer to patterns of contributing factors. . . . They identify deeper characteristics that many superficially different phenotypes have in common.

Cook RI, Woods DD, Miller C.
A Tale of Two Stories: Contrasting Views of Patient Safety.

Chicago: National Patient Safety Foundation. 1998. [42]
Available at: www.npsf.org/exec/report.html.

Harm

Death, or temporary or permanent impairment of body function/
structure requiring intervention.

National Coordinating Council for Medication Error Reporting
and Prevention.
Taxonomy of Medication Errors.
National Coordinating Council for Medication Error Reporting,
and Prevention. 1998. [6]
Available at: www.nccmerp.org/taxo0514.pdf.

High-reliability organizations

Highly complex, technology-intensive organizations that must operate, as far as humanly possible, to a failure-free standard.

Reason J.
Managing the Risks of Organizational Accidents.
Aldershot, UK: Ashgate. 1997. [213]

Hindsight bias

Finding out that an outcome has occurred increases its perceived
likelihood. Judges are, however, unaware of the effect that outcome
knowledge has on their perceptions. Thus, judges tend to believe
that this relative inevitability was largely apparent in foresight,
without the benefit of knowing what happened.

Fischoff B.
Hindsight ≠ foresight: the effect of outcome knowledge on judgment under uncertainty.
J Exper Psycho Human Percept Perform.
1975;1:288–299. [297]

Iatrogenic illness

Any illness that resulted from a diagnostic procedure or from any form of therapy. In addition, we included harmful occurrences (ie, injuries from a fall or decubitus ulcers) that were not natural occurrences of the patient's diseases. However, the term "iatrogenic" should not be construed to mean that there was any culpability on the part of the physician or hospital, or that the illness was necessarily preventable.

Steel K, Gertman PM, Crescenzi C, Anderson J.
Iatrogenic illness on a general medical service at a university hospital.
N Engl J Med. 1981;304:638–642. [638]

Incident

Involves damage that is limited to parts of a unit, whether the failure disrupts the system or not.

Perrow C.
Normal Accidents. Living with High-Risk Technologies.
Princeton, NJ: Princeton University Press. 1999. [66]
(Reprint with new afterword and foreword.)

Incident reporting

A process used to document occurrences that are not consistent with routine hospital operation or patient care.

Cullen DJ, Bates DW, Small SD, et al.
The incident reporting system does not detect adverse drug events: a problem for quality improvement.
J Quality Improvement. 1996;21:541–548. [541]

Individual accidents

Ones in which a specific person or group is often both the agent and the victim of the accident. The consequences to the people concerned may be great, but their spread is limited.

Reason J.
Managing the Risks of Organizational Accidents.
Aldershot, UK: Ashgate. 1997. [1]

Individual errors

Those deriving primarily from deficiencies in the physician's own knowledge, skill, or attentiveness.

Wu AW, Cavanaugh TA, McPhee SJ, et al.
To tell the truth: ethical and practical issues in disclosing medical mistakes to patients.
J Gen Intern Med. 1997;12:770–775. [770]

Isolation

A means [in industry] to separate a process with high probability of failure from other processes to minimize the impact on the products being produced.

Williams E, Talley R.
The use of failure mode effect and criticality analysis in a medication error subcommittee.
Hosp Pharm. 1994;29:331–332,334–336,339. [331]

Lapses

Internal events [that] generally involve failures of memory.

Reason J.
Managing the Risks of Organizational Accidents.
Aldershot, UK: Ashgate. 1997. [71]

Latent failures

Delayed-action consequences of decisions taken in the upper echelons of the organization of system. They relate to the design and construction of plant and equipment, the structure of the organization, planning and scheduling, training and selection, forecasting, budgeting, allocating resources, and the like. The adverse safety effects of these decisions may lie dormant for a very long time.

Reason J.
Foreword.
In: Bogner MS, ed.
Human Error in Medicine.
Hillsdale, NJ. Lawrence Erlbaum Associates; 1994. [xi]

Medical mistake

A commission or an omission with potentially negative consequences for the patient that would have been judged wrong by skilled and knowledgeable peers at the time it occurred, independent of whether there were any negative consequences. This definition excludes the natural history of disease that does not respond to treatment and the foreseeable complications of a correctly performed procedure, as well as cases in which there is a reasonable disagreement over whether a mistake occurred.

Wu AW, Cavanaugh TA, McPhee SJ, et al.
To tell the truth: ethical and practical issues in disclosing medical mistakes to patients.
J Gen Intern Med. 1997;12:770–775. [770]

Medication error

Any preventable event that may cause or lead to inappropriate medication use or patient harm while the medication is in control of the healthcare professional, patient, or consumer. Such events may be related to professional practice, health care products, procedures and systems, including prescribing; order communications; product labeling, packaging, and nomenclature; dispensing; distribution; administration; education; monitoring; and use. [Follows consensus definition by National Coordinating Council for Medication Error Reporting and Prevention]

Cousins DD.
Developing a uniform reporting system for preventable adverse drug events.
Clin Therap. 1998;20(suppl C):C45–C59

Mispractice/malpractice

Physicians also ordinarily do a worse job than juries or judges in distinguishing between honest misjudgments (the currently popular term is "mispractice") and negligent errors (ie, malpractice).

Kapp MB.
Medical error versus malpractice.
DePaul J Law. 1997:1:751–772. [756]

Mistakes

The actions may conform exactly to the plan, but the plan is inadequate to achieve its intended outcome.

Reason J.
Managing the Risks of Organizational Accidents.
Aldershot, UK: Ashgate. 1997 [71]

Misuse

When an appropriate service has been selected but a preventable complication occurs and the patient does not receive the full potential benefit of the service.

Chassin MR, Galvin RW, and the National Roundtable on Health Care Quality.
The urgent need to improve health care quality.
JAMA. 1998;280:1000–1005. [1001]

Monitoring and vigilance failures

Those in which the essence is a failure to recognize or act upon visible data requiring a response.

Cooper JB, Newbower RS, Kitz RJ.
An analysis of major errors and equipment failures in anesthesia management: considerations for prevention and detection.
Anesthesiology. 1984;60:34–42. [38]

Near miss

An event or situation that could have resulted in an accident, injury or illness, but did not, either by chance or through timely intervention.

Doing What Counts for Patient Safety: Federal Actions to Reduce Medical Errors and Their Impact.
Report of the Quality Interagency Coordination Task Force (QuIC) to the President, February 2000. Quality Interagency Coordination Task Force. Washington, DC. [91]
Available at: www.quic.gov/report/index.htm.

Negligence

Care that fell below the standard expected of physicians in their community.

Brennan TA, Leape LL, Laird NM, et al.
Incidence of adverse events and negligence in hospitalized patients. Results of the Harvard Medical Practice Study I.
N Engl J Med. 1991;324:370–376. [370]

Negligent injuries

By definition, in negligent injuries the standard of care and the procedures to prevent injury are well known, as well as the likelihood of serious injury if they are not followed.

Leape LL, Lawthers AG, Brennan TA, Johnson WG.
Preventing medical injury.
Qual Rev Bull. 1993;19:144–149. [144]

Normal accident

If interactive complexity and tight coupling — system characteristics — inevitably will produce an accident, I believe we are justified in calling it a *normal accident,* or a *system accident.* The odd term *normal accident is* meant to signal that, given the system characteristics, multiple and unexpected interactions of failures are inevitable. . . . System accidents are uncommon, even rare; yet this is not all that reassuring, if they can produce catastrophes.

Perrow C.
Normal Accidents. Living with High-Risk Technologies.
Princeton, NJ: Princeton University Press. 1999. [5]
(Reprint with new afterword and foreword.)

Organizational accidents

Comparatively rare, but often catastrophic, events that occur within complex modern technologies such as nuclear power plants, commercial aviation, the petrochemical industry, chemical process plants, marine and rail transport, banks and stadiums. Organizational accidents have multiple causes involving many people operating at different levels of their respective companies.

Reason J.
Managing the Risks of Organizational Accidents.
Aldershot, UK: Ashgate. 1997. [1]

Overuse

When a health care service is provided under circumstances in which its potential for harm exceeds the benefit.

Chassin MR, Galvin RW, and the National Roundtable on Health Care Quality.
The urgent need to improve health care quality.
JAMA. 1998;280:1000–1005. [1001]

Patient safety

The avoidance, prevention, and amelioration of adverse outcomes or injuries stemming from the processes of health care. These events include "errors," "deviations," and "accidents."

Cooper JB, Gaba DM, Liang B, Woods D, Blum LN.
National Patient Safety Foundation agenda for research and development in patient safety.
MedGenMed. 2000:2(4).
Available at: www.medscape.com/MedGenMed/PatientSafety.

Phenotype of an incident

What happens, what people actually do or what they do wrong, what you can observe. Phenotypes are specific to the local situation and context—the surface appearance of the incident.

Cook RI, Woods DD, Miller C.
A Tale of Two Stories: Contrasting Views of Patient Safety.
Chicago: National Patient Safety Foundation. 1998. [42]
Available at: www.npsf.org/exec/report.html.

Potential adverse drug event

An incident in which an error was made but no harm occurred.

Bates DW, Spell N, Cullen DJ, et al.
The costs of adverse drug events in hospitalized patients.
JAMA. 1997;277:307–311. [308]

Preventability

Implies that methods for averting a given injury are known and that an adverse event results from failures to apply that knowledge.

Leape LL, Lawthers AG, Brennan TA, Johnson WG.
Preventing medical injury.
Qual Rev Bull. 1993; 19:144–149. [144]

Risk management

In the context of hospital operations, the term *risk management* usually refers to self-protective activities meant to prevent real or potential threats of financial loss due to accident, injury, or medical malpractice.

Kramen SS, Hamm G.
Risk management: extreme honesty may be the best policy.
Ann Intern Med. 1999;131:963–967. [963]

Root cause analysis

A process for identifying the most basic or casual factor or factors that underlie variation in performance, including the occurrence of an adverse sentinel event.

Joint Commission on Accreditation of Healthcare Organizations.
Conducting Root Cause Analysis in Response to a Sentinel Event.
Oakbrook Terrace, Ill.: Joint Commission on Accreditation of Healthcare Organizations. 1996. [1]

Rule-based behavior

Familiar procedures applied to frequent decision-making situations.

Battles JB, Kaplan HS, Van der Schaaf TW, Shea CE.
The attributes of medical event-reporting systems: experience with a prototype medical event-reporting system for transfusion medicine.
Arch Pathol Lab Med. 1998;122:231–238. [231]

Serious event

One that leads to or prolongs a hospitalization, contributes to or causes death, or is associated with cancer or a congenital anomaly.

Rogers AS, Israel E, Smith CR, et al.

Physician knowledge, attitudes, and behavior related to reporting adverse drug events.
Arch Intern Med. 1988;148:1596–1600. [1600]

Serious outcome

Death, a life-threatening condition, initial or prolonged hospitalization, disability, or congenital anomaly, or when intervention was required to prevent permanent impairment or damage.

Kessler DA, for the Working Group.
Introducing MEDWatch: a new approach to reporting medication and device adverse effects and product problems.
JAMA. 1993;269:2765–2768. [2768]

Sharp end

Where practitioners interact directly with the hazardous process in their roles as pilots, mechanics, air traffic controllers, and in medicine, as nurses, physicians, technicians, pharmacists and others.

Cook RI, Woods DD, Miller C.
A Tale of Two Stories: Contrasting Views of Patient Safety.
Chicago: National Patient Safety Foundation. 1998. [13]
Available at: www.npsf.org/exec/report.html.

Skill-based behavior

Routine tasks requiring little or no conscious attention during execution.

Battles JB, Kaplan HS, Van der Schaaf TW, Shea CE.
Arch Pathol Lab Med. 1998;122:231–238. [231]

Slip

An unintended error of execution of a correctly intended action.

Senders JW, Moray NP.
Human Error: Cause, Prediction, and Reduction.
Hillsdale, NJ: Lawrence Erlbaum Associates. 1991. [28]

System

A set of interdependent elements interacting to achieve a common aim. These elements may be both human and nonhuman (equipment, technologies, etc.).

Kohn LT, Corrigan JM, Donaldson MS.
To Err Is Human: Building a Safer Health System.
Washington, DC: National Academy Press. 2000. [211]
Available at: http://books.nap.edu/html/to_err_is_human.

System errors

The delayed consequences of technical design or organizational issues and decisions. Also referred to as latent errors.

Battles JB, Kaplan HS, Van der Schaaf TW, Shea CE.
The attributes of medical event-reporting systems: experience with a prototype medical event-reporting system for transfusion medicine.
Arch Pathol Lab Med. 1998;122:231–238. [231]

Systems approach

Using prompt, intensive investigation followed by multidisciplinary systems analysis . . . to [uncover] both proximal and systemic causes of errors. . . . It is based on the concept that although individuals make errors, characteristics of the systems within which they work can make errors more likely and also more difficult to detect and correct. Further, it takes the position that while individuals must be responsible for the quality of their work, more errors will be eliminated by focusing on systems than on individuals. It substitutes inquiry for blame and focuses on circumstances rather than on character.

Leape LL, Bates DW, Cullen DJ, et al.
Systems analysis of adverse drug events.
JAMA. 1995;274:35–43. [40]

Underuse

The failure to provide a health care service when it would have produced a favorable outcome for a patient.

Chassin MR, Galvin RW, and the National Roundtable on Health Care Quality.
The urgent need to improve health care quality.
JAMA. 1998;280:1000–1005. [1001]

Appendix Two

A Collection of Web Site Information

The Web sites listed in this appendix discuss patient safety, quality of care, improving care, medical mistakes, medical errors, adverse events, and risk management. Although this is partial listing, many of the sites named here contain links to other sites. More information can be found by searching the Web on key terms such as *patient safety* and *medical errors*.

Specialty

American Academy of Dermatology (AAD)
www.aad.org

The AAD is committed to achieving the highest quality of dermatological care for all individuals. Achievement of this mission requires a dynamic organization to provide excellence in patient care, education, and research; adhere to ethical conduct; and respond to its members and to the public with unification and representation of the specialty.

American Academy of Orthopedic Surgeons (AAOS)
www.aaos.org

The AAOS was founded at Northwestern University in 1933, is a nonprofit organization, and serves as an advocate for improved patient care.

American Academy of Pediatrics (AAP)
www.aap.org

The AAP specializes in the care of infants, children, adolescents, and young adults. AAP believes that children deserve and require the highest quality of health care.

American Board of Emergency Medicine (ABEM)
www.abem.org

The ABEM is dedicated to safeguarding the public by promoting and maintaining the quality, integrity, and standards of training in and practice of emergency medicine, and to improving the quality of emergency medical care for patients.

American Board of Medical Specialties (ABMS)
www.abms.org

"The mission of the ABMS is to maintain and improve the quality of medical care by assisting the member boards in their efforts to develop and utilize professional and educational standards for the evaluation and certification of physician specialists." The ABMS also provides links to other medical specialty areas: see www.abms .org/links.asp.

American Hospital Association (AHA)
www.aha.org

The AHA is committed to improving the health of individuals.

Anesthesia Patient Safety Foundation (APSF)
www.asahq.org/hcfa/apsf.html

Formed in 1985, the APSF is committed to ensuring patient safety. The mission of APSF is that "no patient shall be harmed from anesthesia." The APSF has been successful with its efforts to improve the safety of anesthesia and reduce adverse events.

AnesthesiaPatientSafety.com
www.anesthesiapatientsafety.com

This site "is designed to promote safe anesthesia patient care through public education."

American Society of Anesthesiologists (ASA)
www.asahq.org

The ASA was founded in 1905 and is the primary advocate for all patients who require anesthesia. The ASA is organized to raise and maintain the standards of medical practice of anesthesiology and improve patient care. This site provides links at www.gasnet.org/societies.php.

American Society of Health-System Pharmacists (ASHP), Center on Patient Safety
www.ashp.org/patient_safety

The mission of the ASHP Center on Patient Safety is to foster fail-safe medication use in health systems through the leadership of pharmacists. The center helps pharmacists improve this process through leadership and guidance, professional advocacy, tools and education, alliances and partnerships, and research.

Council of Medical Specialty Societies (CMSS)
www.cmss.org

Founded in 1965 as a nonprofit medical professional association, the CMSS is committed to quality medical care for all patients, improving standards of delivery of care for patients, and studying responses to medical and health care issues. CMSS provides links to other related sites: see www.cmss.org/related/index.html.

Maplecrest Healthcare Systems
www.del-crane.com/html/webres.htm

This site contains links to medical libraries, sources of information, and specialty fields.

MEDSTAT Group
www.medstat.com

"The MEDSTAT Group is a health information company that provides decision support systems, market intelligence, benchmark databases, and research for managing the purchase, administration, and delivery of health services and benefits."

Government

Agency for Healthcare Research and Quality (AHRQ)
www.ahrq.gov

The AHRQ provides information on health care outcomes, quality, cost, use, and access. This information helps individuals make more well informed decisions and improve the quality of health care services.

Centers for Medicare and Medicaid Services (CMS), formerly the Health Care Financing Administration (HFCA)
www.hcfa.gov; www.cms.gov

CMS is dedicated to providing information and service to Medicare and Medicaid beneficiaries.

Department of Veterans Affairs, Office of Congressional Affairs
www.va.gov/OCA /testimony/09fe00PS_USA.htm

This site reports the statement of Thomas L. Garthwaite, M.D., Deputy Undersecretary for Health Department of Veterans Affairs at the VA Patient Safety Program on February 9, 2000, regarding patient safety.

Department of Veterans Affairs, Virtual Learning Center on Patient Safety
www.va.gov/med/osp/cgi-bin /patient.asp

At this site, individuals can browse patient safety lessons gathered from adverse events that may already have happened or that could happen.

Medicare
www.medicare.gov

This is the official site of the U.S. government for Medicare information.

National Committee for Quality Assurance (NCQA)
www.ncqa.org

NCQA strives to improve health care quality for all individuals.

National Forum for Health Care Quality Measurement and Reporting (NQF)
www.qualityforum.org

The purpose of this quality forum is to develop a quality measurement and strategy that covers issues consistent with improvement in health care.

Quality Interagency Coordination Task Force (QuIC)
www.quic.gov

The QuIC was established in 1998, and its mission is ensuring that federal agencies that purchase, provide, study, or regulate health services are working together toward the common goal of quality of care.

General

American Association of Health Plans (AAHP)
www.aahp.org

"AAHP's mission is to advance health care quality and affordability through leadership in the health care community, advocacy and the provision of services to member health plans."

Australian Patient Safety Foundation (APSF)
www.apsf.net.au

The mission of APSF is to provide leadership in the reduction of patient and individual injury in health care delivery systems and to support ongoing research in patient safety and improve patient safety.

Buyers Health Care Action Group
www.choiceplus.com

This site assists its users with finding providers and facilities and with making well-informed decisions.

Catharsis Medical Technology (CMT)
www.catharsismedical.com

The CMT is committed to improving patient safety and improving the quality of care for patients by developing and implementing information technology products that protect patients.

The Foundation for Accountability (FACCT)
www.facct.org

FACCT is a nonprofit organization committed to helping Americans make better health care decisions.

Health Grades, Inc.
www.healthgrades.com

Health Grades is committed to improving health care quality in the United States.

Institute for Healthcare Improvement (IHI)
www.ihi.org

IHI is an independent, nonprofit organization working to increase improvement in health care systems.

Institute for Safe Medication Practices (ISMP)
www.ismp.org

The ISMP is a nonprofit organization that works with health care institutions, practitioners, and agencies to provide education about drug events and their prevention. The ISMP provides an independent review of medication errors that have been submitted, voluntarily, by practitioners.

Institute of Medicine (IOM)
www.iom.edu

The IOM's mission is to "advance and disseminate scientific knowledge to improve human health." The institute provides information and advice on health and science policy to the corporate sector, the government, the professions, and the public.

Joint Commission on Accreditation of Healthcare Organizations (JCAHO)
www.jcaho.org/sentinel/safety.html

JCAHO is dedicated to improving patient safety in health care organizations.

The Journal of the American Medical Association (JAMA)
jama.ama-assn.org

JAMA, begun in 1883, is an international, peer-reviewed general medical journal committed to promoting the science and art of medicine and the improvement of the public health.

The Leapfrog Group for Patient Safety: Leapfrog Initiatives to Drive Great Leaps in Patient Safety
leapfroggroup.org/safety1.htm

The three initial methods purchasers in this group are advancing to improve patient safety are computerized physician order entry, evidence-based hospital referral, and ICU physician staffing.

Medical Errors Preventable
www.abcnews.go.com/sections/living/DailyNews/
medicalmistakes991129.html

This site contains a report by Lauran Neergaard of the Associated Press.

Medical Mistakes Affect Many
archive.abcnews.go.com/sections/living/medmistakes1009

This site contains the text of an article by Claudine Chamberlain on medical mistakes.

MedicalErrorReduction.com
www.medicalerrorreduction.com

This site offers information on medical errors and patient safety. A few of its purposes are to be a place for consumers and providers to learn about patient safety and medical errors; a place for individuals who have been involved with medical errors to share their stories; and a place with links to other sites throughout the world that are working to eliminate medical error and improve patient safety.

Minnesota Alliance for Patient Safety (MAPS)
www.mnpatientsafety.org

The mission of MAPS is to promote the best patient safety through collaboration and support among the participants in Minnesota's health care system.

National Business Coalition on Health (NBCH)
www.nbch.org

"NBCH member coalitions are committed to community health reform, including an improvement in the value of health care provided through employer-sponsored health plans and to the entire community."

National Health Care Purchasing Institute (NHCPI)
www.nhcpi.net

The institute is dedicated to improving the quality of health care, with the goal of helping health care purchasers to save lives, purchase better health care quality, and choose higher quality health plans.

National Patient Safety Foundation (NPSF)
www.npsf.org

The mission of NPSF is to improve patient safety in the delivery of health care. For links to other sites of interest to NPSF, see www.npsf.org/html/web_sites.html.

Pacific Business Group on Health (PBGH)
www.pbgh.org

The PBGH is a nonprofit organization committed to improving health care quality.

Partnership for Patient Safety (P4PS)
www.p4ps.org

"P4PS is a patient-centered initiative to advance the reliability of health care systems worldwide."

Patient Safety Being Left Behind
www.usatoday.com/life/health/errors/cover.htm

This site contains an article on patient safety and medical errors, by Robert Davis and Julie Appleby, *USA Today*.

Voluntary Hospital Association (VHA)
www.vha.com

"VHA was founded in 1977 to support hospitals that wanted to preserve the nonprofit health care philosophy of providing health care to people regardless of their ability to pay."

Name Index

L

LaBar, G., 53, 57
Laffel, G., 81, 99, 172
Laird, N., 9, 30, 32, 55, 57, 80, 81, 98, 99, 112, 172, 265, 268, 277
Landau, M., 195, 198
Landis, J. R., 32
Langa, D. M., 82
Langer, E., 191, 198
Lanier, D., 59, 81
LaPorte, T., 192, 199, 202, 204, 216
Laventurier, M. F., 106, 113
Lawrence, D. M., 119, 123, 135
Lawrence, S. L., 82
Lawry, T. C., 95, 99
Lawthers, A. G., 30, 32, 55, 57, 80, 81, 112, 218, 232, 265, 277, 279
Lazenby, H. C., 32
Leape, L. L., 7, 30, 31, 33, 37, 38, 53, 54, 55, 57, 58, 73, 80, 81, 86, 87, 90, 92, 98, 99, 112, 123, 135, 157, 164, 171, 172, 217, 218, 231, 232, 265, 268, 277, 279, 282
Lee, C. Z., 189, 198
Lee, J., 135
Lehman, B., 108, 109
Leiter, M., 39, 41, 42, 44, 47, 52, 57
Lembcke, P. A., 103, 113
Levering, R., 89, 99
Levi, L., 228, 233
Levinson, W., 60, 80
Levit, K. R., 23, 32
Levy, R., 162, 172
Liang, B., 7, 32, 279
Lipsitz, S. R., 17, 30
Lloyd, J. F., 20, 31
Lloyd-Bostock, S., 58, 82
Localio, A. R., 7, 8, 9, 30, 32, 55, 57, 80, 81, 112, 265
Lusk, E., 81

M

MacKenzie, C. F., 228, 232, 234
Mackersie, R. C., 232
Magi, D., 167, 172
Mainous, A. G., III, 60, 80

Ma'Luf, N., 135
Manning, B. E., 171
Marber, S., 121, 135
March, J. G., 222, 233
Marmor, T. R., 22, 32
Marrin, C.A.S., 173
Mashaw, J. L., 22, 32
Maslach, C., 40–41, 42, 57
Maurer, H., 104, 113
McCormack, J., 118, 135
McDonald, C. J., 128, 135, 157, 172
McGinnis, J. M., 62, 81
McGuire, T. E., 171
McMahon, L. F., 13, 31
McNulty, M., 19, 32
McPhee, S. J., 62, 82, 274, 275
Medalie, J. H., 82
Mendelsohn, R. S., 103, 113
Merrick, N. J., 173
Merritt, A. C., 217, 221, 222, 225, 232
Meterko, M., 48, 56
Meyerson, S., 45, 57
Michaelson, M., 228, 233
Micklethwait, J., 89, 99
Millenson, M. L., 101, 108, 113, 246
Miller, C., 269, 271, 279, 281
Miller, G. C., 60, 80
Miller, W. L., 82
Mills, D. H., 4, 32, 105, 106, 107, 113, 240, 266
Mitchell, P. H., 98
Mohr, J. C., 107, 113
Moore, F. D., 270
Moore, J. D., 125, 136
Moore, P., 86, 99
Moray, N., 64, 82, 281
Moskowitz, M., 89, 99
Mulcahy, L., 58, 82
Munro, A. P., 59, 81, 137, 249
Mushlin, A. I., 98

N

Nader, R., 104, 111
Nagel, D., 221, 234

Subject Index

303

System dynamics, medical. *See* Medical interdependence
System errors: definition of, 282; failure to address, 107; and patient perspective, 110–111
System metaphor, unpacking, idea derived from, 191
System vocabulary, adopting, issues surrounding, 177–178
System-level consequences, 202, 203, 206, 209
Systems: highly reliable, 192–193, 194–197, 208; predictability of, 208; social character of, 193
Systems analysis, 123, 154
Systems approach: categories in, 169–170; definition of, 282
Systems design: in aviation industry, 123; innovation in, 53, 54, 171; and MCOs, 122
Systems failure, internal, manifestations of, 77
Systems management, 124–125
Systems questions, example of, 197
Systems variables, 169–170

T

Targeting research areas, 263
Task load variable. *See* Workload demands
Taxonomy of error. *See* Error taxonomy
Teaching hospitals, laws and recommendations for, 106
Team training, 229
Teamwork, 70, 89, 119, 193–194, 218; surveying attitudes about, 220, 221, 225–226
Teamwork error, 228
Technical complications, 11, *12*
Technical errors, 209–210
Technical uncertainty, 43
Technology, electronic. *See* Electronic technology, use of
Technology-based perspective, 121–122

Technolust, control over, 155
Terminology: commonality in, 130; issues of, sorting out, 256–258; standardization of, 208, 241, 243
Tertiary prevention, 62
Therapies, underuse and overuse of, 94
Therapy-related adverse events, *12*, 38. *See also* Omission, errors of
Third-party payers, values of, 214
Third-party reimbursement, limitations in, 139
Time pressures, manifestation of, *79*. *See also* Workload demands
To Err Is Human: Building a Safer Health System (Kohn, Corrigan, & Donaldson), x, 3, 37, 58, 87, 157, 177, 188, 200, 237–239. *See also* Institute of Medicine (IOM) report
Tolerance: of adverse events, 207, 209, 214; for frustration, 43, 44, 45; of incompetence, 219; zero, 86
Tort system. *See* Malpractice (tort) system
Total Quality Management (TQM), 89
Tracking medication errors, surveying role of, 129
Tradeoffs, 201, 230. *See also* Marginal reliability
Traffic officer analogy, 8
Training: in aviation industry, 123, 192, 218, 224; medical, 218, 228, 229
Transport system, patient, attention to, 180–181
Trauma resuscitation, observation of, 227–228
Trauma simulators, 228, 229
Treatment: naturalistic view of, 167–168; validation of, 132
Trending, 143, 145, 150
Triangulation, 263
Trust: creating environment of, 98, 141, 146, 149; eroding, 92, 148; restoration of, in health plans, 134; in risk management, 137–138